HYPNOSIS IN CRITICALLY ILL PATIENTS: ANXIETY, DEPRESSION AND SUICIDAL BEHAVIOR.

Ps. Gabriel Pérez Almoza

© 2024 Pérez Almoza
First English Edition
First Spanish Edition, 2020
Clinical Hypnosis Center of Chile
Nueva Providencia 2211 Of.818, Providencia

Phone: 2 22325119 - 569 98792141

Santiago de Chile.

www.hipnosisclinica.cl

All rights reserved.

This publication may not be reproduced in whole or in part, or recorded in, or transmitted by any information retrieval system, in any form or by any means, mechanical, photochemical, electronic, magnetic, photocopying, photocopying or otherwise without the prior written permission of the Publisher.

GABRIEL PÉREZ ALMOZA

To my family, mother, wife and children

ACKNOWLEDGMENTS

To Rafael Segundo Bestard Bizet who showed me the human sensitivity with which our patients should be treated.

To Luis Enrique Cortés Pérez for introducing me to the wonderful world of Therapeutic Hypnosis.

To my great friend, tutor and teacher Alberto Erconvaldo Cobián Mena who shows me that believing in Hypnosis is one of the best alternatives for the treatment of different mental disorders.

To Juan Cristóbal Schilling Fuenzalida, for his dedication and support in the preparation of this book, for opening the doors and giving his trust.

FOREWORD

According to the World Health Organization, depression is the leading cause of disability in the world. Depression, despite its multiple causes, is based on hopelessness and helplessness, leaving patients with a sense of paralyzing helplessness, and usually perceiving their future as dark, uncertain and distressing.

In my work as a clinical hypnotherapist psychologist I seek first of all to listen and understand those problems that afflict our patients, most of them associated with emotions of pain, sorrow and anguish. As we are attending people in our consultations we learn about the most diverse internal ghosts that live within each of them. Childhood traumas, loss of loved ones, sexual abuse, infidelity, sexual dysfunction and a myriad of events that make their lives a nightmare.

Each patient comes to our sessions with a general purpose, which by the way is the same as the vast majority of people; to be happy, to have a peaceful life, to achieve inner peace.

This is how each of us as therapists, with the tools that the university gives us in their training, in addition to others acquired over time and experience are put at the service of the patient.

Sometimes, without realizing it, we are trying to guess the possible actions and changes of our patients in case of doing this or that intervention. In this way we seek to read their future, clearly with the instruments we have access to.

The big problem is that many times, our clinical intervention criteria is not always so precise and clear, especially with patients with deep depressions. Our objective will be then that the patient can achieve a greater emotional balance and that his life is more bearable, but in no case that this worsens and that our patient thinks or executes an action of suicidal nature.

One way of seeking our internal peace of mind as professionals and safeguarding the patient's integrity will generally be to refer the patient to a psychiatrist for consultation, or to request the patient's urgent hospitalization with family members. But even so, we do not always have great clarity in knowing how much risk there is that our patient commits suicide.

I do not know if physicians are prepared for the death of a patient, perhaps oncology specialists or terminal patients are, but as clinical psychologists we must avoid and be attentive to any sign that the patient presents us in relation to ideation or attempt to take his or her own life. The death of a patient by suicide significantly affects the family, friends and even the therapist. It fills us with doubts about whether there was something we should have done, said or asked that could have changed that hard and definitive determination.

Hypnosis as a treatment tool has an important ability to empower people in a wide variety of ways; however, the use of hypnosis in the treatment of depression has historically been discredited for unfounded reasons. The result has been a glaring dearth of clinical and research literature on the subject.

Gabriel Perez's book gives us more light on how hypnosis can contribute in patients with depression, in a generous text, providing concrete and relevant information. The text is divided in an easy and clear way, favoring a quick reading.

Another aspect to highlight is related to being the first Spanish-speaking author to deal with this topic of such relevance as depression and the risk of suicide. Together with Professor Michael D. Yapko's book "Hypnosis and the Treatment of Depressions", Perez's book is a perfect complement as a guide for health professionals trained in hypnosis and its approach to depressed patients and thus can contribute to the decrease of the painful statistics on suicides.

Cristóbal Schilling Fuenzalida
Director of the Clinical Hypnosis Center of Chile.

HISTORICAL-LOGICAL ANALYSIS

There are several considerable enigmas in human life, suicide being one of them. No one really knows why a human being deprives himself or herself of life, and the assertion that there is no valid reason to assume such behavior does not stand up to any objection. Unraveling the mysteries that emanate from suicidal behavior is part of science. [1]

Suicide is a major health problem, a real existential drama of man, recognized since ancient times in the Bible, in the Christian Era it is considered a sin, condemned by the Church every individual with suicidal behavior. [2]

At the beginning of the 20th century, studies on suicide began with two main currents, the Sociological, represented by Dorkheim, and the

Psychological, presented by Meninger and Freud, which involved different mechanisms inherent to the psyche. [3]

The World Health Organization defines a suicide attempt as any action by which the individual causes injury to himself, regardless of the lethality of the method employed and the actual knowledge of his intention, it should be seen in the light of current knowledge as a failure of the individual's adaptive mechanisms to his environment. [1]

It is caused by a current or permanent conflict situation that generates a state of emotional tension or as a consequence of various causes, a concept that provides a comprehensive and dialectical assessment of the factors involved in the event. [1-3]

Suicidal behavior is defined elsewhere as any act committed to the detriment of the perpetrator, with varying degrees of lethal intent and includes attempted and completed suicide,[6] although it describes a continuum from suicidal ideation to suicide, where suicidal behavior encompasses completed suicide, attempted and threatened suicide as well as the ideation of the act, with specific thoughts and ideas, called by some authors parasuicide and pre-suicidal syndrome. [4]

Suicidal ideation is understood in this study as an alteration defined as a constant in the categories that make up suicidal behavior in general. It is undeniable the presence of ideation for the suicidal act either from the implicit elaboration to the consummated act.

Suicide attempt and suicide are the two most representative forms of suicidal behavior; although they represent a journey from suicidal ideation to suicide. Suicidal ideation ranges from the idea of the difficulty of living to transient, prolonged, impulsive, planned and permanent suicidal ideation.

Parasuicide or attempted suicide is defined as any action by which the individual causes injury to himself regardless of the lethality of the method used and the actual knowledge of his intention. Suicidal intent is conceived in two ways: when the subject performs an act of self-harm with the threat of death, but his final intention was not to take his own life, and when he fails in his attempt to kill himself once the act has been performed. [5]

These have many meanings and whatever their degree of lethality, special attention should be paid to them: they are the living sample to know the truth about the characteristics and causes of people adopting self-destruction. The consummated suicide causes great impact in the society, where from remote times the most diverse answers are determined and it is the origin of infinite speculations, philosophical discussions and great literary production. [7]

Suicide is a multifactorial cause in which biological, psychological and social factors intervene, being considered as the expression of a "failure" in the adaptive mechanisms of the subject to the environment, caused by a situation of current or permanent conflict that generates a state of emotional tension. [8]

It results from a complex fact that requires for its understanding of a comprehensive interdisciplinary approach that encompasses the influence of individual, social and family factors that induce to attempt the self-destruction of a person; behaving as the conscious act of self-induced annihilation, best understood as a multidimensional discomfort in a needy individual that delimits a problem, for which the act is perceived as the best solution.

It is important to know that during the stage of adolescence and young adulthood, systematic changes occur in human beings related to the attitudes assumed by young people in the psychological, physiological, sociocultural and biological aspects, where independence is acquired, family detachment is achieved and some behaviors are generated that have a negative impact on the family and social environment, which produces unhealthy lifestyles such as suicidal behavior that affects their quality of life. [9, 19]

Adolescents who attempt or commit suicide are characterized by different risk factors for this behavior, among which are cited:

-Coming from socially disadvantaged and educationally impoverished backgrounds.

-Exposure to adverse family situations that condition an unhappy childhood.

-Those with psychopathology including depression, substance abuse and dissocial behavior.

Low self-esteem, impulsivity, hopelessness, broken loves or socioeconomic problems.

-Lack of communication with parents, hopelessness and abuse, among other aspects, which limit the active social participation of adolescents, prevent them from satisfying their most basic needs and restrict their freedom. [20]

On a practical level, the suicide attempt or even the very idea of suicide sometimes represents a first order urgency due to the risk of recidivism and consummation of the act. From a theoretical point of view, the field of adolescent psychopathology is poorly placed within the classical psychiatric variables. In fact, the exact number of suicide attempts among adolescents is not known, since most of them are covered up by the subject himself and his family. [21-25]

There are different methods of taking one's own life, the soft or less lethal ones such as the ingestion of psychotropic drugs, toxic substances, etc., and the hard or lethal methods such as hanging, precipitation from heights, burns, section of blood vessels, use of firearms and others. In general, men use the hard methods, which is why they have a higher mortality rate.

CLINICAL EPIDEMIOLOGICAL BEHAVIOR

Worldwide, suicide rates have increased 60% in the last 45 years and 90% of the cases are associated with depression and substance abuse. Every year one million people commit suicide and every day in the world 1110 individuals commit suicide and as many attempt it, of which only one tenth succeed, regardless of geography, culture, ethnicity, religion, socioeconomic status, among others.[26]

Across Germany nearly 10,000 people took their own lives in 2008, an extreme behavior more frequent among men than among women. The figures are chilling: every 40 seconds someone in the world takes his or her own life; in Germany almost 9,500 people committed suicide in 2008, but this is only a small fraction of those who attempted suicide, some 38,000.

In France about 1000 suicides concern children and adolescents with a prevalence of 70% in men. The most common method used by the latter is hanging, while women resort to taking medication. France has one of the highest rates of this type of death, ranking fourth after Finland, Austria and Luxembourg, according to a 2008 study by the Institut de

Santé et de la Recherche Médicale (Institute of Health and Medical Research).

In 2010, the World Health Organization reported that the global suicide rate was 16 per 100,000 population. In the Americas, suicide has reached large proportions during the last decades and has become a major health concern.

In 2013, suicide claimed 842,000 lives, being the tenth leading cause of death, it is estimated that there have been an average of 10 to 20 million suicide attempts which have failed in their ultimate goal, to end the life of the person, but have caused from minor to severe injuries, where young females predominate. [27-30]

Suicidal behavior is highly prevalent worldwide. Developed countries report high mortality rates due to this behavior and offer data that rise above 30 suicides per 100,000 inhabitants and in some exceed 40; unsuccessful attempts are an indicator of around 10 for each completed suicide.[31]

In the United States of America, according to a report by the Center for Disease Control, it is the twelfth leading cause of death. In 2010, a total of 38,364 deaths by suicide were reported, which were associated with economic causes, showing an increase in the numbers of this scourge. A year earlier, it was the seventh leading cause of death for men and the sixteenth leading cause of death for women. [32]

Suicide is the third leading cause of death among adolescents and young adults between 15 and 24 years of age and it is estimated that from 1999 to 2010 it has generally increased in the 35 to 60 age group, with an increase of approximately 30 to 50 percent for males and 60 percent for females.

In Latin America, the highest incidence of suicide occurs in young people between 15 and 19 years of age, although Canada, the United States, Cuba and Venezuela have the highest rates. It has also been found to be between the third and fourth leading cause of death in the 15-44 age group and accounts for 6.5% of all deaths in this age group. [38]

Uruguay has high rates for the region (10 per 100,000 inhabitants). Internationally, it is estimated that attempted self-harm is 10 times higher than suicide; with drug use there are elements of predisposition to aggressive behavior.

In Cuba, the first reports of suicide date back to the time of Spanish colonization and are referred to by *Fray Bartolomé de las Casas*, about groups of individuals who preferred to hang themselves rather than endure the torments and calamities of colonization, as did the African slaves. [33-35]

The first epidemiological report in Cuba dates from 1940, where data on suicide was analyzed and processed from 1902 to 1971 and found a higher incidence in older men with a predominance of hanging, but not in women with the use of fire. [38]

The social development achieved by Cuba has made it possible to make a qualitative leap in the health system, which is shown in an increasingly comprehensive care of the problems that affect the health status of men and their families. The incidence of suicidal behavior has had a tendency to decrease in recent years, although it continues to be a problem that increases in localities of the national territory. [5,38]

In the 1960s, with a rate of 15.4 x 100,000 inhabitants and as part of the profound social changes brought about by the triumph of the Revolution, Psychiatry Services were integrated into the National Health System (SNS), seeking total coverage of the population, equity in their provision, and the integrity of promotion, prevention, care for harm and rehabilitation actions.

Its focus is shifting towards primary health care (PHC) and the biometric model is gradually replaced by the biopsychosocial and salubrious model.

It relies on the political will and the participation of the organized community. At the National Forum on Hygiene and Epidemiology in 1974, the problem of psychiatric epidemiology was addressed for the first time. Since 1980, the crude rate has remained above 20.

Until 1982, when the highest rate in the last 30 years occurred: 23.2 per 100,000 inhabitants, which represents deaths by suicide, 4% of the deaths that year. A national investigation was carried out, as a result of which the National Program of Attention to Suicidal Behavior was launched.

Today it is the ninth leading cause of death, according to data provided by the National Office of Statistics and Information of the Republic of Cuba and behaves as follows:

-In 2008 for 1377 cases.

-In 2009 for 1472 cases.

-In 2010 for 1557 cases.

-In 2011 for1529 cases.

-In 2012 for 1495 cases.

-In 2013 for 1490 cases. [5]

These data are edited after the year, in the first months of the following year, for a better closing and tabulation of the national data obtained. It should be clarified that the incidence of suicide has been decreasing, and changes are noted in the reports of the main causes of death between 10 and 19 years of age. Despite this reduction, it is a health problem.

Suicide is the fourth leading cause of death in the 15-49 age group, with a rate of 17.6 per 100,000 population. [5]

The National Statistics Directorate of MINSAP in Cuba reports approximately six attempts for every deceased person and a slight increase in suicide attempt rates between 10 and 14 years of age, which is very worrying, demonstrating that it continues to be one of the main causes of death.

Addressing it should be a priority for the improvement of psychosocial issues in the lives of the general population. In 2006, the provinces in the country that had the highest suicide rates for all ages are: Havana with 15.9; Pinar del Río with 15.2; Granma with 12.3 and Holguín with 14.1 x 100 thousand inhabitants.

The province of Guantánamo, at the end of 2010, had a mortality rate of 12 per 100,000 inhabitants and 1,305 attempts were made.

In Holguín province suicide behaves as the eighth cause of death, according to data provided by the National Statistics and Information Office of the Republic of Cuba behaving as follows: Year 2017 for 187 cases.

Year 2009 for 147 cases.

Year 2010 for 175 cases.

Year 2011 for 169 cases.

Year 2012 for 164 cases.

Year 2013 for 197 cases. [38]

In Cuba, self-inflicted injuries in the period from 2016 to 2017 for the age group of 10 to 19 years, ranked third with 29 and 32 deaths respectively.

In Banes in 2018, 18 patients died from this cause. This evidenced an initial increase in both the number of people who attempted against their lives; as well as those who lost their lives.

The assessment carried out at the "César Fornet Fruto" University Polyclinic on this behavior in adolescents allows the author to note the alarming increase in self-injury in these cases.

In 2015, 5 patients died from this cause and 57 attempted against their life, among them 21 adolescents, in 2016, 38 attempted suicide, among these, 17 adolescents, 3 patients died from this cause. In 2017, 3 patients committed suicide and 68 attempted suicide, of which 23 were adolescents. In 2018 the figures were: completed suicides 10, suicide attempts: 44, of which 15 are adolescents.

The above points out that suicidal behavior is associated with common preventable risk factors related to lifestyle and way of life, which is why it is necessary to work on the basis of the objectives set forth in the National Program for the Prevention of Suicidal Behavior.

The first priority is to prevent the first suicide attempt, its repetition and consummation, placing in the hands of medical and paramedical personnel a working instrument to achieve the reduction of deaths and thus comply with the health indicators desired by our ministry and thus improve the mental health of the population. There is a lack of knowledge in the psychotherapeutic management of suicidal ideation in adolescents.

For these reasons and in response to national research guidelines. The scientific idea arises of how to contribute to the psychotherapeutic management of pediatric patients with suicidal behavior so that the scientific and clinical community can obtain a functional tool for the adequate treatment of this health problem.

SUICIDAL BEHAVIOR AND ITS DIFFERENT APPROACHES.

At the end of the 19th century, the modern era in the interpretation of suicide began with the work of Durkheim and Freud. Durkheim takes a sociological approach to suicide and argues that it is the result of the strength or weakness of society's control over the individual. He defines three types:

Altruistic suicide: It is literally requested by society, due to its culture, norms and customs. The individual has no other honorable option left. To continue living would be an ignominy. It is the case of the harakiri among the ancient samurai.

Selfish suicide: In this case the person has few ties with the community; they are people who live alone, have no family or social group or institution to relate to. There are practically no social demands for the individual.

Anonymous suicide: It is produced by a sudden rupture in the usual relationship between society and the individual.[2]

Blumenthal and Schneidman state that suicide is explained by the sciences from different angles, with sociological and psychological approaches predominating. Today, there is a consensus that none of these theories in isolation is capable of providing a complete explanation of this phenomenon, which is in fact multifactorial, being determined by psychological and social elements.

The influence of biological factors is not ruled out and they conceptualized suicide as: "the human act of self-induced annihilation". Suicide attempts are much more frequent than suicides with an epidemiological confirmation of 30 to 1, where drug intoxications occur repeatedly.

The vulnerability to make a suicide attempt increases significantly when a person has lost control of his or her emotional impulses, especially when this takes place in an environment of hostility, where significant behavioral or emotional symptoms develop in response to one or multiple psychosocial factors. [4,55]

These events include processes related to the individual's age, occupational, personal, family, health problems - illness or death of a family member.

Elements for assessing suicidal behavior.

The World Health Organization considers taking into account the following elements for the correct evaluation of the patient with Suicide Attempt.

a) Suicidal ideation (sporadic-persistent).

b) Determination (suicide as a possibility-straightforward decision to commit suicide).

c) Suicidal plan (developed suicide plan-increased risk: availability of means for suicide increases risk).

d) Loneliness (lack of social and family support increases the risk).

e) Alcoholism (its consumption limits the capacity for self-control and may favor suicidal behavior).

f) Social difficulties (marginality, unemployment, lack of expectations, lack of belonging group) and lists the different factors associated with this behavior.[40-43]

<u>Within suicidal behaviors, the following should be highlighted:</u>

a) Suicidal ideation.

b) Suicide planning: how, where and when to carry out the self-destructive behavior, the place and sometimes even the day chosen.

c) Parasuicide: it is a generally non-fatal act, which has increased in recent times, especially in adolescent or young women. It is impulsive and involves the use of drugs.
d) It is frequent in those people with abrupt mood changes or with personalities of antisocial characteristics. There are depressive symptoms in 10% of cases and an environment of social disorganization is observed.
e) Suicide: its main characteristic is that it is fatal and premeditated. It is more common in males, with a normal pre-morbid personality. There is depression in 70% of cases and social isolation is frequent. [9]

The motivation that leads the individual to make a suicide attempt, which he or she finally succeeds or fails, is what is defined as motive, regardless of the method used, which refers to the way or means by which these people decided to take their own life, whether hard or soft.

Suicide attempt, together with suicide, are the two most representative forms of this behavior, although not the only ones. Unfortunately, there are many texts that only take into account these two aspects, which are the most serious ones, and not others that, if detected and taken into consideration in a timely manner, would prevent both from occurring.

The full spectrum of suicidal behavior is made up of the ideation of self-destruction in its different gradations: threats, the gesture, the attempt and the consummated act. [9, 56]

Forms of presentation.

Suicidal ideation encompasses a wide range of thoughts that may take the following forms of presentation:

- The desire to die ("Life is not worth living", "I should just die", etc.).

- Suicidal representation ("I imagined that I was hanging myself").

- The idea of self-destruction without planning the action ("I'm going to kill myself", and when asked how he is going to do it, he answers: "I don't know how, but I'm going to do it").

- Suicidal ideation with an undetermined or unspecific plan ("I am going to kill myself in any way, with pills, throwing myself in front of a car, burning myself").

- Suicidal ideation with adequate planning ("I have thought of hanging myself in the bathroom while my wife is asleep"). It is also known as a suicidal plan.

Extremely serious.

All these manifestations of the ideation of self-destruction should be explored, if the patient does not manifest them, since communication and open dialogue on the subject do not increase the risk of triggering the act, as erroneously considered, and is a valuable opportunity to initiate its prevention. [3]

Suicidal threats are verbal or written expressions of the desire to kill oneself and should be taken into account, because it is a common mistake to think: "He who says it, does not do it" or "He who kills himself, does not warn that he is going to do it". When the threat occurs and one has the means available for its realization, but without carrying it out, it is considered by some as a suicidal gesture (having the pills in the hand without taking them) and should never be minimized or valued contemptuously as "a boast". [2]

It is considered that the attempt is more frequent in young people, in the female sex, and the most used methods are soft or non-violent, mainly the ingestion of drugs or toxic substances.

First of all, it must be considered that these traits are individual, since what for some is a risk element, for others does not represent a problem at all. In addition to being individual, they are generational, since factors in childhood may not be the same in adulthood or old age. On the other hand, they are generic, since those of women are not similar to those of men. There are those that are common to all ages and sexes, which are undoubtedly the most important. [18]

Factors associated with suicidal behavior.

Children and Adolescents:

Individual predispositions: presence of mental health disorders: depression, previous suicide attempts, substance abuse, drug use, learning problems, impulsivity, school failure, disabling diseases, vulnerability to humiliating elements, disengagement from study and/or work, involuntary institutionalization, alteration of sexual identity, ascription to groups with disruptive behaviors.

Family: parental violence, sexual abuse, alcohol and drug abuse, isolation, history of suicidal behavior, accepted suicidal behavior, death or separation of family members, family rejection, ease of means that facilitate suicidal behavior, poverty, family neglect.

Community: Socio-economic deterioration of the community, little or no access to sports, recreational, cultural activities, etc., high incidence of alcoholism and other addictions and accepted suicidal behavior.

Public Health in Cuba has a preventive character whose objective is to prevent the appearance, development and prolongation of diseases, whether communicable or not. To this end, it has to favor the maintenance of health or put barriers to the risk factors that determine the occurrence of the disease, as well as to achieve early diagnosis, treatment and rehabilitation to avoid and limit the disability that can cause it. [9]

Suicidal behavior is associated with common preventable risk factors related to lifestyle and lifestyle, so an integrated fight against them must be carried out.

In the work context of the Basic Health Team, which is nothing more than the community, the family doctor and nurse, once they detect the risk, are able to implement health education actions with the intention of modifying inadequate behaviors, always with intersectoral management. [27, 57]

ERRONEOUS AND SCIENTIFIC APPROACHES TO SUICIDE

There are several erroneous criteria regarding suicide, suicidal people and suicide attempters, which must be eliminated if you wish to collaborate with this type of people. Let us list some of them, not all of them, of course, and we will expose the scientific criteria that from this moment must prevail in you to be able to make effective your help in the prevention of suicide.

Wrong criterion: He who wants to kill himself does not say so.

Scientific criterion: Of every ten people who commit suicide, nine of them clearly stated their intentions and the other hinted at their intentions to end their lives.

Wrong criterion: He who says it does not do it.

Scientific criterion: Everyone who commits suicide expressed with words, threats, gestures or behavioral changes what would happen.

Wrong criterion: Those who attempt suicide do not wish to die, they only make the boast.

Scientific criterion: Although not all suicide attempters wish to die, it is a mistake to label them as boastful, since they are people whose useful coping mechanisms have failed and who find no alternatives except to attempt against their lives.

Wrong criteria: If he really wanted to kill himself, he would have thrown himself in front of a train.

Scientific criterion: Every suicidal person is in an ambivalent situation, i.e., with a desire to die and a desire to live. The method chosen for suicide does not reflect the death wishes of the person who uses it, and providing him/her with another method of greater lethality is qualified as a crime of aiding the suicide (helping him/her to commit suicide), penalized in the Penal Code in force.

Wrong criterion: The subject who recovers from a suicidal crisis is in no danger of relapse.

Scientific criterion: Almost half of those who went through a suicidal crisis and consummated suicide, carried it out during the first three months after the emotional crisis, when everyone believed that the danger had passed. It happens that when the person improves, his movements become more agile, he is in a position to actually carry out the suicidal ideas that still persist, and before, due to inactivity and inability of agile movements, he could not do it.

Wrong criterion: Everyone who attempts suicide will be in that danger for life.

Scientific criteria: Between 1% and 2% of those who attempt suicide succeed during the first year after the attempt and between 10% and 20% will complete it in the rest of their lives. A suicidal crisis lasts hours, days, rarely weeks, so it is important to recognize it for prevention.

Wrong criterion: Everyone who commits suicide is depressed.

Scientific criterion: Although every depressed person is likely to make a suicide attempt or suicide, not all those who do so present this maladjustment. They may suffer from schizophrenia, alcoholism, character disorders, etc.

Wrong criterion: Everyone who commits suicide is mentally ill.

Scientific criterion: The mentally ill commit suicide more frequently than the general population, but one does not necessarily have to suffer from a mental disorder to do so. But there is no doubt that every suicidal person is a suffering person.

Wrong criterion: Suicide is inherited.

Scientific criterion: It has not been demonstrated that suicide is inherited, although several members of the same family can be found who have ended their lives by suicide. In these cases, what is inherited is the predisposition to suffer from a certain mental illness in which suicide is a main symptom, such as affective disorders and schizophrenia.

Wrong criterion: Suicide cannot be prevented because it occurs by impulse.

Scientific criterion: Every person before committing suicide evidences a series of symptoms that have been defined as pre-suicidal syndrome, consisting of constriction of feelings and intellect, inhibition of aggression, which is no longer directed towards other people, keeping it to oneself, and the existence of suicidal fantasies, all of which can be detected in due time and prevent them from carrying out their intentions.

Wrong judgment: Talking about suicide with a person at this risk may encourage him or her to commit suicide.

Scientific criterion: It has been demonstrated that talking about suicide with a person at such risk, instead of inciting, provoking or introducing the idea in his head, reduces the danger of committing it and may be the only possibility offered by the subject for the analysis of his self-destructive intentions.

Wrong approach: Approaching a person in suicidal crisis without proper preparation for it, using only common sense, is detrimental and wastes time for a proper approach.

Scientific criterion: If common sense makes us assume a posture of patient and attentive listening, with a real desire to help the person in crisis to find solutions other than suicide, prevention will have begun.

Wrong criterion: Only psychiatrists can prevent suicide.

Scientific criteria: It is true that psychiatrists are experienced professionals in detecting the risk of suicide and its management, but they are not the only ones who can prevent it. Anyone interested in helping this type of person can be a valuable collaborator in its prevention.

Wrong criterion: The subject of suicide should be treated with caution because of the socio-political problems it causes.

Scientific criterion: The issue of suicide should be treated in the same way as other causes of death, avoiding sensationalist news and those manipulations that provoke the imitation of this behavior. On the other hand, suicide as a cause of death is observed in countries of different socioeconomic regimes, from the highly developed to those with scarce resources, as it responds to different factors, such as biological, psychological, social, psychiatric and existential factors.

THE PERSON AT RISK OF SUICIDE AND ITS MANAGEMENT

I will now present several ways to handle a person with the possibility of committing a suicidal act and alert the reader that any method, as long as it is authentic, harmonizes with the personality characteristics of the person using it, is used by those who believe in its effectiveness and aims to prevent the consummation of such an act, can achieve good results in suicide prevention.

I. In the case of any patient at risk of suicide, the first thing to be evaluated is whether the subject can take responsibility for his or her life or is not in a position to do so. This implies considering who this person has been, who he/she is now, comparing him/her with the data previously collected, in order to make clear the differences, if any, that may precipitate a suicidal act. This also includes the search for the healthy and intelligent part of the patient, with whom we must work to reduce the probabilities of actually carrying out the self-injurious intentions.
In parallel, it should be explored what other resources in the family and environment are available to prevent the person from attempting or

committing suicide. Just as the healthy part is assessed, the sick part of the individual should be assessed, i.e., his degree of mental disturbance: whether or not he is deprived of his mental faculties and whether or not he is able to participate constructively in his self-help.

And also if this person has real reasons to continue living, so it is necessary to find out if he/she is married, if he/she has children, if he/she works and feels satisfied with what he/she does, if he/she has friends or belongs to any political, religious or fraternal organization, etc., his/her state of physical health and sense of well-being, among other questions.

After this analysis between who this subject was and who he is now, at this time of risk, potentially suicidal people can be divided into three categories:

First category: People unable to take responsibility for their lives. This category includes those who have very little reason to continue living, such as the elderly alone and without family to take care of them and who have other added suicidal risk factors, such as painful, incapacitating illnesses that require several surgical interventions, poor economic situation, sadness, crying, suicidal ideas, threats to take their own lives, frequent alcohol intake, marked insomnia, incipient dementia, etc. Individuals with severe psychiatric illnesses such as schizophrenia, mood disorders, depression and complicated alcoholism; the insane and the moderately to severely mentally retarded, as well as those physically ill with cancer or AIDS, and those suffering from severe chronic pain.

Finally, children must remain among the people who are not responsible for their lives, because, really, they are not.

Second category: Persons with partial responsibility for their lives. This category includes those who suffer from the diseases in the previous section at a certain point in their evolution, when it is possible to maintain contact with the physician, they are manageable in their family environment and their current symptoms are not serious.

Also included are the mildly mentally retarded, uncomplicated alcoholics and, of course, adolescents, who, although they are not sick like children, require, unlike them, not guardianship, but guidance and advice.

Third category: This category includes persons with full responsibility for their lives, such as those with personality disorders, minor or non-serious psychiatric illnesses, physical illnesses with psychological repercussions but with lucid consciousness, situational problems without symptoms of serious alterations in psychic functioning, and, of course, adults without psychiatric disorders.

With each of these categories a different intervention should be made, according to the following diagram:

The main purpose of this management is to check whether the subject is able to cooperate with the care of his own life and with those who want to help him to take care of it. The less cooperation there is, the more precautions should be taken because the more likely it is that the suicidal act will be carried out, regardless of the degree of responsibility for his or her life.

II. This variant is to confront the person who has made a suicide attempt. It consists of trying to answer a series of questions in conversation with the potential suicide. Let's go on to enunciate them:

1. Who was this person before the attempt on his or her life?

From the answers to this question it is possible to know the factors that increase the risk of committing suicide:

- Previous psychiatric illness.
- History of suicide attempts.
- Social maladjustment.
- Inadaptation at work.

- Family maladjustment.

- Coming from a psychiatric family or having psychiatric relatives.

- Coming from a family of suicides or suicide survivors.

Who is this person now?

The comparison between the answers to the previous question and this one can give a closer approximation to the risk of suicide, because the greater the differences between what a person was and what he/she is, the greater the risk of suicide may increase. This also includes the current clinical picture, i.e., the symptoms presented, and it is the planned suicidal idea that is the most dangerous due to the proximity to the execution of the act; the family, work and social maladjustment in the present, the factors that triggered the suicide attempt, among which family and partner conflicts and associated physical illnesses stand out.

3. Is its lethality high?

Here the answers should guide us on the method used, because although any in certain circumstances can cause death, the so-called hard methods, such as hanging, fire, precipitation from elevated places created by man or natural, section of large vessels, submersion and others, are more dangerous. With regard to the circumstances, special attention should be paid to those who choose places of difficult access, where the chances of rescue are minimal, although suicides have been performed in front of television cameras and millions of viewers.

4. What does the patient say?

This question tries to verify what the suicidal ideation fits in with: whether there is a purpose to die or the act is attributed another meaning such as the desire to show others how big their problems are, escape from an intolerable situation, request for help, etc. The presence of a suicidal plan substantially increases the danger of repeating it successfully, as well as the distorted ideas about reality, the classic "nonsense" as relatives say, that when they have as a theme supposed guilt, self-reproaches, miseries, tragedies, calamities, incurable diseases, etc., entail a high risk of suicide.

5. What is the healthy part of the subject?

The answer to this question is of strategic importance since the definitive management of the subject's suicidal crisis depends on it. The different situations that may arise range from people with hardly any psychic disturbance to those who are seriously disturbed, from those who have a reasoned critique of what has happened to those who consider suicide as the only possibility.

6. What can this subject hold on to, besides me, to keep on living?
This is of great human, fraternal and solidarity value, because, in addition to our help, we must seek support from children, spouses, co-workers, neighbors, etc.

7. What else can I do for this person?
Their response allows for a review of what has been done so far, which has consisted mainly in the assessment of suicidal risk. From now on, efforts should be concentrated on directing the person with suicidal attempts, suicidal threats, planned or unplanned suicidal ideas, to receive qualified care, which can be provided by family physicians, psychologists, psychiatrists, crisis intervention units of general hospitals, etc. This objective of bringing the individual in suicidal crisis closer to health centers is fundamental, and if he does not go to them, a home visit can be requested to the family physician, if he has not already done so as part of his duties.

8. Have I done everything?

As can be seen, this is an incisive question that complements the previous one and seeks to mobilize all available resources, including family, friends, neighbors, community, institutions, organizations and everything necessary to confront a subject with suicidal intentions.

<u>Never leave the person alone in a suicidal crisis.</u>

III. Another variant for the management of the person at risk of suicide.

The first thing to do when a person confides in us his suicidal ideas, is to TAKE IT SERIOUSLY, giving the required importance to the situation, because many make the serious mistake of considering those who attempt suicide as blackmailers, manipulators, that they are acting crazy, that it is a theater or a show. If they think this way, they will never be able to understand or help a presumed suicidal person.

A second step in this management is to try to understand the subject, the motives he/she had to try against his/her life, and to achieve this, it is very important to listen with real interest to what he/she says, carefully, attentively, thus facilitating the release of emotions and feelings which fulfills a cathartic, emetic function, with the consequent relief, even if momentary, but relief nonetheless. All of the above will favor the relationship with him and the help you wish to offer.

Thirdly, we must try to facilitate the individual's own search for solutions to his current problems, for realistic and possible alternatives, since in times of crisis these are substantially reduced, and feelings of self-destruction predominate. It is not convenient to set oneself up as the supreme judge of the subject's acts or to want to take responsibility for his life if he is in a position to do it himself.

The fourth is to banish from your thinking the false idea of minimizing the reason why a person might attempt suicide with expressions such as: "He won't do it because what is happening to him is not a reason to take his own life". For you or another individual without suicidal risk, such a motive may not trigger such an act, but for the individual at risk, a similar motive may precipitate it.

The fifth thing you SHOULD NEVER DO is to challenge him, suggesting methods of greater lethality than he has used in the case of being a survivor of a suicide attempt, such as: "And if you wanted to die so badly, why didn't you throw yourself in front of the train? and the subject had only ingested tablets of a short-acting anxiolytic; or "Just kill yourself once and for all, you have bored me" or "You don't kill yourself at all, don't be doing paperwork", these expressions should be abolished from our lexicon and criticize whoever utters them because, evidently, he does not know the hostility that this type of person generates in him.

Lose the fear of dealing with suicidal people, who are usually able to establish a good relationship with you, are in great need of being listened to and want to continue living with only minor changes in their lives. And never forget that if you intuitively feel that the subject is in suicidal crisis and may commit suicide, try by all means to direct him/her to a medical center for specialized treatment.

IV. When faced with a potentially suicidal person, it is necessary to take into account our own opinions and points of view regarding those who attempt suicide, which may range from outright rejection, considering them cowards, to full justification, labeling them as heroes.

It is not prudent to assume, when facing them, neither one position nor the other. Individuals who attempt or wish to attempt against their lives are neither cowardly nor brave, since cowardice and bravery are qualities of character that cannot be quantified by the capacity of human beings to deprive themselves of their lives or not. These people have failed in their reactive-adaptive capacity, they have failed in their useful mechanisms of adaptation to the vicissitudes of life, and as happens in any case of crisis, they are desperate, confused and with an ambivalent mixture of feelings.

In this situation it is very useful to serve as an "orthopedic model" for this type of individuals, giving them frequent support, helping them in the analysis of their problems and difficulties, facilitating their participation in the search for solutions together with other family members, fellow students or co-workers, in order to reduce as far as possible the recurrent feelings of loneliness so frequent in suicidal people.

It is a good technique for helping them not to try to convince them how wonderful it is to be alive, how good life is and other similar conversations, because they are not capable of thinking that and far from helping, it may increase their feelings of inefficiency, uselessness, handicap, because they feel unable to enjoy the benefits of living. In this sense, it is more useful to specify in detail what they say about their lives and why they consider that they are meaningless and it is better to die, since the mere expression of these opinions could bring them some relief, besides allowing us to know how they think.

It should not be forgotten for a moment that people with this risk have very limited alternatives to solve problems and the most common is suicide, so it is of great importance to know them and evaluate how realistic they are, and if the danger is high; from that moment on they should not be left alone.

Finally, spend some time with them to make them understand the other non-suicidal options for solving problems that would cause suffering to those close to them if they died, as well as those who wish to help them, not forgetting to mention the sources to turn to for mental health care if the desire for self-harm persists, in which case you are the person to approach them.

V. A somewhat complicated variant of handling these people at risk of suicide is that in which the first thing to do is to diagnose the meaning of taking one's own life for those who wish to take their own life or have tried to do so. Not all self-harmers have a real desire to die. The effects resulting from self-injury without the intent to kill are called self-inflicted harm and, as I have already pointed out, they can have different meanings, which are necessary to determine in order to manage these persons more effectively.

Many inflict harm on themselves in order to avoid physical pain, a fundamental symptom caused by a certain disease. It is not necessary the evidence of the same, but they can attempt against life because of what is to come, as is the case of incurable diseases. In this situation, the essential thing is to assure the individual that there are fundamental medicines in sufficient quantity to cope with this contingency and, if this fails, there are other techniques to put an end to the pain, available in specialized institutions.

Some people wish with suicide to attack other loved ones, so it is useful to discuss the subject of aggressiveness and how to make it socially useful, because it is not bad to be aggressive, but to make a bad use of it. A boxer who is not aggressive is not a good sportsman, because in all combat sports aggressiveness is fundamental. And even in these cases it cannot be used willy-nilly, but in an intelligent way that results in victory. The same must be done in everyday life.

Others react in this way to the loss of a valuable relationship, and in these cases they should be reminded of other losses that have preceded the present one, relate past and present states of mind and assess to what extent this situation has regained the same meaning of past experiences. But now he is an adult and is expected to face them in a more mature, more realistic, less dependent, less harmful way for him and those around him.

Many of those who attempt against their life are indicating that they have made their debut in a certain mental illness of importance, with the need for specialized attention as soon as possible due to the danger of consummating suicide, and the orientation towards a psychiatric clinic for their diagnosis, treatment and follow-up of their evolution by competent professionals becomes urgent.

Some of them resort to suicide trying desperately to ask for help because they are faced with a problem they are unable to solve on their own because it is beyond their ability to cope. In these cases, the best thing to do is to remove them from the situation if possible by changing their environment, hospitalization, etc., to teach them other ways of coping and to ask for support from as many people as possible who are involved with this individual and the solution to their problem. Finally, there are those who wish to take their own life in order to get out of an overwhelming difficulty such as a conflictive and difficult relationship, a precarious socio-economic situation, unavoidable responsibilities for which they are not prepared, etc. A good alternative in these cases is to provide emotional support to the subject, human warmth and to assess how stress can be reduced to relieve their tensions.

VI. One way to help people at risk of suicide is to know how they feel at that moment. It is common for them to feel terribly alone, with no one interested to understand them. In many cases, the isolation in which they immerse themselves facilitates these feelings. They often consider life to be meaningless, assume that other people would feel better if they did not exist and that it is preferable to be dead.

They feel pessimistic, they believe that nothing has gone, is going or will go well in their lives, that they are a calamity and their difficulties have no solution. There are not few desperate people whose suicidal fantasies in their minds become more firm and convincing with each passing minute. But coupled with this they also feel a great desire to go on living if certain changes were to occur, if they were to be given a little help.

It is convenient to eliminate the mistaken criterion of not being able to help them with simple common sense, because they only need to be listened to and assisted. When faced with a person who confides in you his or her desire to commit suicide, I suggest the following:

- Do not be alarmed to receive this information, but always take it seriously.

- Encourage her to confide in you about her problems and how they make her feel.

- Speak as little as possible so that the voice of the person suffering always predominates.
- Touch the person, as skin-to-skin contact facilitates communication (e.g., light manual pressure on the forearm while inviting the person to vent).
- Do not use yourself as an example, or talk about yourself and your personal experiences.
- Do not give her the solutions that were good for you, as they may not work for her at all.
- If you do not feel confident in what you are doing, ask for help. It is not advisable to handle people at risk of suicide alone when there is insecurity.
- Stay with her until the danger has passed, which may be manifested by her being able to verbally express criticism of suicidal thoughts when her mood improves, and she is more relaxed, calm, cooperative, and interested in daily activities.
- If suicidal risk persists, take the subject for specialized psychiatric care.
- Try it again when anyone else confides in you about their suicidal intentions and it will work out better than the first time, as it did for all of us who have dedicated ourselves to suicide prevention.

MANAGEMENT OF A PERSON WHO MAKES A SUICIDE ATTEMPT OUT OF REVENGE OR BLACKMAIL

The suicide attempt for revenge or blackmail, is made by people with abnormal traits in their character, who intend, through this act, to punish others, to put them in evidence as guilty of their suicidal act and, in the case of death, to make them responsible for their death.

People who make this type of suicide attempt have relatively often assumed the role of victims in their interpersonal relationships or that of manipulators of others. In most cases, they intend to punish someone very closely related to them, such as a father, mother, spouse, boyfriend, girlfriend, etc., for something they did or did not expect them to do or did not do and they wanted it to be done.

Almost always, the time elapsed between the alleged problem or motive and the suicide attempt is short: minutes, hours, rarely days, so that the other person, and with him/her the others, can realize the close relationship between what happened and the suicidal act. Sometimes they may leave farewell notes or contradictory messages such as the following: "Don't blame Fulana for what I do, but since what she did to me I can't think of anything else but death."

Conventional approaches to the management of suicidal behavior.

1. It is convenient to let this person know that no human being is guilty nor can make another commit suicide: it is the subject himself who attempts suicide who chooses the method and he himself who puts it into practice. When an individual causes the death of another, it is no longer a suicide, which by definition is killing oneself, but a homicide. In this sense, it is said that suicide is the homicide of oneself.

2. He must understand that the responsibility for the suicide attempt lies with the subject himself, for not having adequate control of his impulsivity and inadequate management of his hostility, for not having learned to cope with complex situations and choosing abnormal coping mechanisms.

3. The analysis of who punishes whom with such an attempt must be made. Undoubtedly, the person to be punished will continue to live, although with a certain degree of guilt, the closer the emotional bond that united them. However, the most severely punished is the one who attempts it, because in the first instance he may lose his life or affect his health; he may lose the trust of his loved ones who will begin to treat him

with fear, pity or compassion, but not as a normal person; he will be the comment of the neighborhood, because they will think that he is not in good mental health.

It should be emphasized that the alleged punisher, from that moment on, will have difficulties in knowing why the relationship with him or her continues, whether it is because there is still love or because they are afraid of his or her reactions, in the case of the partner, one of the most frequent cases. You should also understand how much your future possibilities of affective stability and of finding a normal partner are limited, since it is difficult to maintain lasting bonds with someone who has attempted suicide to take revenge on a loved one.

4. We must invite him to modify his abnormal way of loving, because it is a serious mistake to believe that "he who loves you well will make you cry"; when you really love you do not blackmail your loved one or make him the object of any revenge or manipulation.

5. He needs to understand how essential it is to modify his way of being and doing, that is, his behavior, if he intends to be as balanced a person as possible. And one of the characteristics of this one is that he does not self-aggregate to blame others for what he does against himself.

6. The subject is the only one responsible for his life and also for his death, and in that death by suicide, the main role will be played by his own way of being, by no other person, and he must be made to understand this.

7. Emphasize the need to differentiate between the motive for an event and its cause. The motive for a suicide attempt by revenge or blackmail can be anything, an upset, the breakup of a relationship, a frustration, etc. But the cause of this abnormal behavior is the subject himself, with his abnormal way of handling situations.

8. Finally, it is necessary to invite him to make use of the good, adult and responsible part of his personality, which will surely prevent the realization of acts of this type, an evident sign, without a doubt, of immature character traits.

MANAGEMENT OF A PERSON WHO MAKES A SUICIDE ATTEMPT OUT OF FEAR

This type of suicide attempt is made by those who try to avoid a very feared situation, hence the importance of defining what it is. There are moments that generate diverse fears in the generality of human beings, such as wars, epidemics, famines, natural catastrophes. Some only generate it in certain people, but not in others, because they are circumstances that usually do not produce this type of emotion. These are the so-called phobias, irrational fears of difficulties, objects or animals and multiple things depending on their origin.

There are other very feared setbacks, not because of the situation itself, but because of the consequences derived from it in certain cultural contexts. Let us take for example the case of a teenage girl in a home, brought up with rigid moral principles among which virginity is the main currency of honor, and losing it means being a dishonor for her and the family.

Let's suppose that this adolescent, out of love, curiosity, curiosity or any other valid reason for herself at that moment, has sexual relations with her boyfriend, that fear of facing the consequences of her act may lead her to attempt suicide to avoid paternal or maternal anger, the scolding of relatives, gossip and comments, etcetera. In these cases, family members react with a range of intermingled effects, which can range from anger to physical aggression, because they feel that the adolescent has humiliated them in front of everyone.

<u>In circumstances of this type, I suggest the following handling:</u>
We must make parents understand how limited their criteria of a good and honest daughter is, because a good daughter is a good daughter because she is studious, sociable, kind, self-sacrificing, loving, respectful, truthful, punctual, and a whole series of personal qualities that surely their daughter has and they have not stopped to value, because they are only interested in whether or not she is a virgin.

2. Because of the rigidity described above, which has played the role of a separating wall, there are difficulties in parent-daughter communication, and prevented the adolescent from communicating what had happened and opting to attempt suicide.

3. There has been a deficient sexual education in the adolescent and in the parents, which favored premarital sex at this stage of life.

4. The adolescent should understand that very fearful situations are equally fearful for all human beings and the rest can be classified as very important, important and unimportant, and help her to classify hers according to this new criterion, which excludes fear.

5. Family members and the adolescent should know that each problem should be given its due value. Neither overvalue nor undervalue it, and it is advisable to bring it to the attention of others who are not immersed in it and who may have a more realistic view of it. The family doctor, the psychologist, the psychiatrist, the priest or pastor, a good friend, etc. can be used for this purpose.

6. The message must reach them that at important moments such as the one referred to above, is when you prove to be a father or mother to your daughter, because it is preferable to have a daughter who is not a virgin than to have a daughter who is dead or a survivor of a suicide attempt.

7. The adolescent must understand that at important moments you show your parents that you are a daughter by trusting them. At first they will not react as expected, but if you go about your life as usual, fulfill your obligations, give them time for reflection, everything will return to normal.

8. The family must analyze that the problems that arise in its bosom are not necessarily to create chaos and disorganization. Many times the crises in the family contribute to the individual growth of its members from the emotional point of view and this is translated in more solid and realistic bonds. In this new dimension, the family to be helped will be urged to function.

Finally, there are multiple situations that generate suicidal acts, but all of them will have intolerance as a common denominator, unilateral fear motivated by cultural factors that, in spite of us and yours, still persist.

MANAGEMENT OF A PERSON WHO MAKES A SUICIDE ATTEMPT OUT OF DESPERATION

Suicide attempts due to despair occur in the course of circumstances with great emotional repercussions in individuals with low tolerance to frustrations; most frequently after disappointments in love, although it is not exclusive to them, nor are they the only ones in which it can occur.

For the management of this type of suicide attempt, the following questions are first asked of the subject in question:

- Does everything always have to go right in life?
- Do things always have to turn out the way we think and want them to?
- Are human beings vaccinated against failures, disappointments and disappointments?
- Are disappointments, frustrations and all the problems that happen to us to commit suicide or to face them, suffer and give them a solution, if they have one, and continue living with that experience gained?

It would then be very useful to reflect with the individual:

Not everything in life has to go right and that does not constitute a tragedy. He is the one who does it, because it did not turn out the way he wanted and because he has not yet learned to face adverse situations. A person who wants to be balanced has to be able to recognize his mistakes, to let go of valuable possessions or give up something when circumstances require it.

2. He is not the only one who has suffered love failures, frustrations, disappointments, loss of loved ones, in short, the various problems that occur, because they are part, precisely, of that which is called LIFE and must be LIVED, even if they are painful and very frequent.

No human being is immunized against failure. There are vaccines for multiple infectious diseases and our country is in an advanced position in this field of medicine, but there is not and will not be created an anti-disgust, anti-failure, anti-problem vaccine. It should never be said "I cannot get upset", "I cannot get upset", when to be fair it should be said "I have not learned to get upset", "I have not learned to get upset". In fact, there are those who from early times of their lives were always indulged in all their whims by their loved ones and being adults, firmly believe that the rest of the people who are not their relatives, are obliged to please them as they did. And that most of the times will not happen, and will cause in the subject the unexpected confrontation and the consequent discomfort.

In order to be balanced, he must avoid being annoyed unnecessarily, avoid annoyances because he takes them into account and prevents them; but he must not avoid them either if they arise, because in the course of life he must learn to face them.

4. Failures, disappointments in love, make people feel bad, frustrated, disillusioned, pessimistic, irritable or any other type of psychic state that is not usual, but not abnormal either, since it is the logical response to a painful and unpleasant event that has happened to them.

If you want to be balanced, you will suffer from your discomfort but you will continue to do, perhaps with less efficiency and creativity, what you were doing before the suffering: work, raise children, study, etc. You can ask for advice from your family doctor, psychologist, psychiatrist, priest or pastor or simply from a person you trust. All this is normal.

Now, if he wants to complicate his own life, he will do just the opposite: not being able to bear to be suffering, he will start to stop doing the things that can help him to reduce this suffering. He will then begin to neglect his work, his children and his family, shutting himself away.

He will not seek medical help and if he does, he will not fully comply with the therapeutic indications, nor will he confide his problems to others who could help him, and it is in these moments of loneliness, more apparent than real, that these suicidal acts occur.

5. It is essential that you grieve and try to continue to function as normally as possible, learning from everything that has happened and trying to ask yourself what your involvement has been in order to avoid making similar mistakes in the future. If you want to be balanced, you must be able to realize when you have stopped meaning to someone what you meant before. That is always sad and painful, but it is not the end of the world. We are still who we are but without that creature.

A person who wants to complicate her life will think that she did everything right, perfectly, that the other person is to blame, that she was played with, deceived, manipulated, used and without this other being and the conflict that limits her world, everything will be over. Children, family, studies, work, friendships, are not, for her, part of her world and she must be reminded that they are.

6. We must help her to find alternatives other than suicide when facing painful situations, since it is a definitive solution to temporary discomfort.

MANAGEMENT OF THE FAMILY OF A SUICIDAL PERSON

From a certain age, which ranges from approximately seven to ten years old, all normal human beings know that they have to die. However, in spite of this, death always affects, to a greater or lesser extent, those who continue to live, and therefore the way in which one dies becomes even more important, especially if that death is by suicide, violent and unexpected in most cases.

In this regard, it has been pointed out that "the person who commits suicide puts his or her psychological skeleton in the emotional closet of the survivors who have to deal with negative feelings, thoughts about their possible involvement in the suicide or what they failed to do to prevent it".

The cause of death that generates the most guilt, hostility and stigmatization is suicide. Therefore, when facing the family of the suicidal person, the first thing is:

- Consider the degree of shock and what immediate resources are available to the family for emotional support.

- Detect feelings of guilt and responsibility for what happened.

- Detect possible suicidal thoughts, threats and other related behaviors among the deceased's family members.

- Help the family to recognize that the suicide was related to the possible illness of the individual and not to a fault of theirs, as it has been proven that relatives of suicides are at risk of similar behavior by various mechanisms, among which imitation plays its role.

It is convenient to consider that the classic mourning reaction, in the case of the suicide's relatives, is catastrophic in its manifestations.

In the first phase of shock, marked sadness is evident among family members who had a close relationship with the suicidal person, and coexists with physical symptoms, such as jumping stomach, precordial pain, hypersensitivity to noise, feelings of unreality, shortness of breath, loss of energy, appetite and sleep disturbances. The shock phase is followed by a phase of rage, which can be directed against everyone, the doctors who attended the individual, the subject himself, the suicidal person, God, etcetera.

This phase is followed by the guilt phase, in which anguish for not having foreseen the outcome, unfulfilled longings of the suicide, unresolved differences in relationships with the deceased, possible motives that contributed to the fatal outcome, repetitive thoughts and memories of the deceased are notorious. Finally, the reorganization phase allows the survivors to redirect their psychic energies to new motivations if the bereavement is satisfactorily resolved.

Some claim to recognize the phases of grief and not act immediately. In my experience, based on an effective doctor-patient-family relationship, I start the health actions at the funeral itself, limiting myself at those moments to allow the manifestations of pain and grief and even stimulating them in those family members who try to maintain excessive control over their emotions, always taking care to bring the voice of reason where the voice of affection predominates. At this time, the greatest emotional support is given to those who were most affectively linked to the suicidal person.

In the following days we will work with the family to establish differences between expected and unexpected deaths such as suicide, so that they understand how devastating this type of death is for the survivors, and to prevent them from making others go through the traumatic experience they are going through. Another important aspect is to establish what I have called "prioritizing" the grief, that is, to establish a hierarchy of mourners, and to prevent the usurpation of grief by other family members who are not the most affected, but because of certain personality characteristics, behave as if they were the ones who are suffering the most. This procedure should not be applied if there is not a solid relationship with the relatives and a deep knowledge of the links between them and with the deceased, in order to achieve in this way the solidarity of the rest of the family and to provide emotional support to the "prioritized mourner", without the others feeling their feelings minimized, and to increase their altruistic attitudes.

As for the guilt often felt by the survivors of a suicide, it is possible to handle it depending on the degree of responsibility that the deceased may have had for his life. Thus, if the suicide was carried out by a subject with no or only partial responsibility for his life at that time, we make the relatives understand that:

- Guilt is a common phase we all go through when a loved one dies, regardless of the cause; it lasts for a certain period of time during which the individual constantly questions what he or she did or did not do to make the events happen. This is very normal.

- There are diseases, such as the one suffered by this person, in which suicide, although it occurred at that particular moment, could have occurred much earlier and if it did not happen, the care and attention provided by the family had a lot to do with it. Suicide in these diseases is like fever in tonsillitis, it is always present and is not easy to avoid when the person has little or no responsibility for his or her life.

- The suicidal person himself would not have wished to suffer from the illness that led to his suicide, nor the family, nor the doctor, nor the psychologist, nor the psychiatrist. If the suicide had full responsibility for his life, the family is made to understand the following:

- People, when they have a certain way of being, or certain traits in their character, become their own most dangerous enemies.

- The family member is asked: How could you avoid this, and usually responds with those ideas that reflect guilt for what happened, that is, what he/she did not do or did wrong. The relative is listened to carefully and then asked: For how long were you going to be able to avoid what happened? It is possible that he/she will answer with a time limit, after which the following question should be asked: And then, how were you going to avoid the suicide if he/she continued to be that way and had no interest in changing?

If you have not yet understood the message that you want to give her not to feel guilty for what happened, you reason as follows: What is my mother's fault if now, when I finish talking to you, I attempt suicide?

Don't you realize that I am an adult, I do what I want and no one can stop me?

To do that, my mother would have to chain herself to me, sleep with me, bathe with me, go out with me, and that is impossible. Assuming that all that could be done for a while, life would have no quality for her and no quality for me. On the other hand, if she stops being chained to me I may attempt suicide, so she would have to spend her whole life that way, which is an absurdity.

Then another question: Who is taking care of you and me so that we do not commit suicide? Obviously, no one should be responsible for the life of another, unless it is a child, a seriously mentally ill person who is unable to discern between right and wrong, an insane person who has lost all understanding, or a severely mentally retarded person who has never had any.

A last resource can be to ask the relative if he instilled in him the idea of suicide, if he provided him with the means to carry it out, which will surely be answered in the negative. Then, he/she is assured of knowing everything he/she has done to modify his/her way of being, how much advice he/she has given him/her and everything he/she has suffered because of the character of the deceased.

It is more difficult to handle when the guilt is based on real events, such as, for example, that there are family members who attempted suicide prior to the loved one's suicide. In such cases it is not wise to try to remove all the guilt, as this may be perceived as a deception or as an attempt to console the loved one without sufficient reason to do so. It is useful to know the following in relation to this phenomenon:

- The imitative effect of suicidal behavior is recognized. In 1841, William Farr stated: "There is no fact better established than the imitative effect in suicidal behavior". In our days, this effect is related to the handling of the subject by the mass media and the sensationalist news about suicide. The family history of this behavior is always cited as a risk factor and to subtract or deny its importance, knowing this, would expose its lack of authenticity to the person in crisis, who has a special sensitivity to detect when distorted information is given.

- This type of person we are talking about needs to feel guilty, but not totally. He tolerates a part of the guilt that belongs to him and is grateful to be allowed to carry it and continue to live with dignity.

Taking into account these two aspects mentioned, we will make the following observation: "You, it is true, had tried against his life and that logically makes you feel guilty for the suicide of your relative and I consider that this background could have influenced. But if you stop to reflect, he had characteristics in his way of being very different from yours.

From whom did he learn them? We do not know. Just as we cannot determine from whom you learned these things, neither can we say that not loving your life was learned from you, solely and exclusively.

But, in addition, you notice when someone else is doing something wrong and you do not blindly imitate it merely because you witness it or know it happened. In other words, if you know what is good, regular and bad, you don't have to imitate the latter unless you want to, because no one is fatally obliged to imitate the bad when they can try to imitate the good.

How do I see things, then? In my opinion, you did something wrong some time ago, which may have influenced in some way what happened to your loved one, but that is not the cause of the suicide, because this type of behavior is caused by the conjunction of multiple factors and never just one of them. In this particular case, the greatest weight was constituted by his abnormal character traits, which not only caused his death but also led him to have difficulties in school, marriage, with friends, at work, etc.".

Once the relative of the suicidal person with a history of the same attempt has been assisted, it is useful to take certain measures of a general nature that facilitate the elaboration of grief and, therefore, its evolution within normal limits. These measures are:

- Remove photos of the deceased from places where the family frequently gathers. When the bereavement has been resolved, you can place one where you consider it appropriate, since it will no longer be remembered with the affective intensity of the first days. In the meantime, it is better to have some place to go specifically for that and not where the image is found just by passing by.

- Do not carry photos of the deceased with you (wallets, purses, identification documents, medals, etc.).

- Remove your personal belongings by storing them in a safe place, but not visible to the naked eye.

- Modify the room of the deceased or the place where he/she was staying.

- Not attending the cemetery frequently.

- Continue to dress as you always have. If there is a tradition of wearing mourning, do not try to prevent it.

- Allow children to continue to live their daily routine, i.e., play, watch children's programs on TV, etcetera.

- Do not forget that the adolescent has his own way of experiencing his grief for what has happened and does not have to show it in the same way. Even if you see him laughing at certain moments, he suffers as much as you do, don't forget that.

- It is advisable to talk to children about what happened, and always relate suicide with madness (even if it is not true), as this association may reduce the possibility of imitation, "the madman is the one who commits suicide and I am not, therefore, I do not commit suicide".

Ways to manage suicidal behavior in the health area.

The public health approach has strategies for suicide prevention:

- Conduct mental health campaigns, screening in schools, early diagnosis of drug abuse, depression and stress.
- Conduct specific suicide prevention programs and avoid stigmatization of suicidal behavior.
- Control access to the means to commit suicide. There is evidence that controlling gun ownership decreases the suicide rate, as does controlling the use of drugs and pesticides. Other measures may include fencing off high-rise bridges and windows in tall buildings.

Support for the media to tailor information to prevention: Training of journalists in handling information on suicidal behavior, as the media can play a proactive role in helping to prevent suicide.

Suicide prevention involves a series of activities ranging from providing the best possible conditions for the education of children and young people, effective treatment of mental illness and control of risk factors.

It is essential to help people with suicidal behavior to get out of the crisis, and to stop thinking about suicide as a solution, the systematic work of the health team is essential due to the high representation of professionals at that level, as they are able to modify attitudes, behaviors, change the perception of environmental stimuli and thus modify the dysfunctional cognitions that play such an important role in the psychological mechanisms of suicide. [20]

THERAPEUTIC PROPOSALS FOR SUICIDAL BEHAVIOR.

At all times in which suicidal behavior and its different clinical manifestations are studied and treated, some authors try to propose intervention programs, but without defined or standardized achievements that allow to alleviate this phenomenon and reduce its incidence and prevalence in the world population.

There are protocols that only allow a description and characterization of suicidal behavior to define a diagnosis. They do not allow to treat its manifestations from the psychotherapeutic clinic nor to prevent its repetitiveness. [18]

According to *Vicente Martín Pérez* in his proposal "Suicidal behavior. Intervention protocol", he states that: The training of the emergency psychologist in on-site assessment skills, in social skills, in active listening, in establishing empathy, in emotional management and containment, in negotiation strategies. [53]

In short, emotional and cognitive connection skills increase the likelihood of modifying physiological and cognitive responses, and by varying these antecedents, the suicidal person's pro-life operants change.

This research leaves half-heartedly the intentions of dealing with the phenomenon of suicidal behavior from a psychotherapeutic perspective.

The objective lack of a theoretical positioning that allows to know techniques, resources and objectives that provide conclusions in favor of the adequate management of this behavior without enabling the subject to stop manifesting clinical expressions or a personological maturation that prevents a later relapse. [11]

It is pertinent to point out the need to design methodologies from a psychotherapeutic foundation, which with a scientific character, demonstrates the associated symptomatological suppression, an adequate modification of behavior towards suicidal behavior and consequently the personological structuring that allows the appropriate elaboration of frustrating or conflictive situations that trigger in some subjects the self-injury as a response.

In Cuba there is a program that sets out a methodology for action in the National Public Health System for the prevention, control and follow-up of suicidal behavior. The methodological scheme lacks the explicit exposition of the resources in the Psychotherapeutic order for the adequate treatment of this behavior.

The explanation of diagnostic guidelines that stratify suicidal behavior only allows to know it and not to give a timely solution in a psychotherapeutic perspective. The current scientific literature shows a void in this regard, which means that health services do not have structured psychotherapeutic resources for the management of this phenomenon. [3, 7, 9]

HYPNOSIS: CONCEPTS AND PRACTICAL APPLICATIONS.

Definitions of Hypnosis as a state:

According to the American Psychological Association (APA) in 2014, The Executive Committee Division 30 prepared the following official definitions related to hypnosis:

Hypnosis: a state of consciousness involving focused attention and reduced peripheral awareness, characterized by an increased responsiveness to suggestion.

Hypnotic induction: procedure designed to induce hypnosis.

Hypnotizability: The ability of an individual to experience suggested alterations in physiology, sensations, emotions, thoughts or behavior during hypnosis.

Hypnotherapy: The use of hypnosis in the treatment of a medical or psychological disorder or concern.[10, 58]

While there are substantial variations in the theoretical understanding of these phenomena, the above definitions were created in the interest of simplifying communication about hypnotic phenomena and procedures within and between the fields of research and practice, and are intentionally, and to a large extent, atheoretical.

According to *Cobián Mena Alberto E.1997*. "Hypnosis is a special state where it is possible through the word or another stimulus, always potentiated by it and in a repetitive way, to create a special state in the human mind that reduces to the minimum expression the volitional processes and allows the full manifestation of cerebral potentialities that in the waking state and by defensive neurophysiological mechanisms are not manifested in an active way".[12, 13]

According to *Rodríguez Sanchez Pedro Manuel, 2011. Hypnosis is:* "Mode of waking consciousness, in which the focus of attention predominates and which is a state potentially susceptible to develop in all human beings by the technically designed influence of speech, gestures, symbols and expectations through a process of conditioning, which produces, maintains and evokes a special type of excitation of the cerebral cortex of the person who receives them, and this allows the arrival at a more subconscious temporal mode of functioning of the brain, in which the characteristics of the motor, vegetative, sensory, thinking, behavioral, and electrical brain activity change essentially, which manifests itself neurophysiologically in a demonstrable and very characteristic way. This process has an eminently psychological induction, technically designed and intentionally structured in the specialist's discourse, which produces in the receiver objective and regular responses not observed in other states of consciousness, which unobjectionably characterize hypnosis in its different stages of depth." [14]

Theoretical model of the genesis, nature and maintenance of the hypnotic process.

Genesis:

The hypnotic process is generated by the effect of the content and rhythm of the suggestions in the process of communication with the patient with all the psychological processes that take place in it, the word acts as a stimulus that is conditioned during the hypnotic induction, it provokes

temporary neurophysiological changes that give rise to a waking consciousness modality with its own characteristics, which we have named:

Mode of subconscious functioning of the brain in hypnotic state. The conditioning process in the initial stages would follow the known regularities of this process in habitual wakefulness, but, we postulate that from the middle stage, this process would take place under the neurophysiological changes that are being established and that would give it sui generis characteristics.

Evocation:

Communication, psychological processes, suggestions, gestures, words, as already conditioned stimuli, constitute clues that are anchored to the state reached and can easily reinduce it on subsequent occasions without having to go through the initial stages of the process again.

Maintenance:

The more inductions are made, the more the conditioning of the state reached is strengthened (Principle of reinforcement). Communication maintains the modality of consciousness reached, but this has autonomy and independence from the word, so it can be sustained temporarily in the deep stages without communication if the suggestions so indicate.

Temporality: The mode of consciousness that is reached is easily reversible to habitual wakefulness by suggestions or spontaneously with the passage of time.

Divisions of the Nervous System in which objective phenomena of hypnosis are observed in the human being.

- In the sensory systems.

- In the motor system.
- In the vegetative system.
- In the upper nervous system.

Characteristics that support the concept of hypnosis as a modality of the waking state of consciousness:

- In behavior and electroencephalogram (EEG).
- Regularity of hypnotic phenomena.
- Repetitiveness of hypnotic phenomena.
- Similarity of hypnotic phenomena among randomly selected subjects, without previous experience or reference to the hypnotic process.
- Temporariness of the state.
- Neurophysiological bases: vegetative, behavioral and bioelectrical.[15, 16, 62]

Proposed definition of hypnosis as a psychotherapeutic technique.

For the present research, hypnosis is understood as a proposal of the author; without being a concept or definition in itself, but a construction of knowledge that allows structuring hypnosis in the clinical context as a psychotherapeutic tool in the following way:

"Therapeutic hypnosis is a method that conditions a specific state of consciousness which is understood as a modality of the waking state, possible through the word or other stimulus, always <u>creatively and repetitively</u> potentiated by it, it creates a special state in the human mind that <u>intentionalizes the expression of volitional processes</u> and allows the full manifestation of cerebral potentialities that in other states are impossible and due to defensive neurophysiological mechanisms are not manifested in an active way, which is <u>improbable without the will of the experiencing subject</u>, making the level of depth reached and the positive expressions in mind-body health dependent on it". [17, 18, 59]

This construction, which aims to define hypnosis as a psychotherapeutic modality for research purposes, is undoubtedly the most accurate approach as a proposal to intervene in suicidal behavior.

The creativity and repetitiveness that is pointed out conditions that the hypnotic state is stable in time as well as the depth reached. Where the intentional expression of the volitional processes allows the therapist to make an ethical and adequate use of each moment of the treatment according to the objectives defined for it.

The will of each research subject is fundamental for the fulfillment of the objectives to be set at each moment of the research. It is necessary to point out that even when the therapist has a high level of expertise in the use of the hypnotic technique, it depends on the patient's will at the first moment of the induction for the achievement of the same in its different levels of depth as well as the benefits in therapy.

The therapeutic hypnosis and the treatment of anxiety and depression as disorders associated with suicidal behavior:

Hypnosis is an effective tool in the treatment of anxiety and depressive disorders, because it allows to quickly achieve deep states of calm and well-being that reduce the feeling of anxiety and provide immediate relief without the possibility of altering the psychological past and future times. [11-13]

Studies have been conducted in which the authors compared a cognitive-behavioral intervention involving cognitive restructuring and in vivo exposure for public speaking anxiety with an equivalent treatment in which relaxation was replaced by hypnotic induction with suggestion.

Hypnosis was shown to have superior efficacy to other modalities when used as an adjunct to cognitive-behavioral therapy. [52, 53, 60, 61]

With hypnosis you can work more directly with the emotions, with that unconscious part of the mind, and thus facilitate the modification of those exaggerated reactions of fear, worry, anxiety, sadness. That are associated to situations or concrete stimuli or to more general or indeterminate contexts, or even not conscious, as it can be the case of a generalized anxiety or some types of panic attacks or specific depressive reactions.[60, 61]

KEY CONCEPTS AND DEFINITIONS.

Protocol: According to the Diccionario de la Real Academia Española: "Detailed sequence of a process of scientific, technical, medical, etc. performance."

hypnosis: From Eng. *hypnosis,* and this from Gr. ὑπνοῦν *hypnoûn* 'to numb' and *-sis* '-sis'.

1. f. A state produced by hypnotism.

Definition: Proposition that clearly and accurately states the generic and differential characters of something material or immaterial.

Concept: Idea conceived or formed by the understanding. [36]

Determination of variables for the study:

As a dependent variable to Suicidal Behavior where anxiety, depression and self-esteem are manifested as altered emotional states associated with it and were evaluated by means of the Trait-State Anxiety Inventory, Trait-State Depression Inventory, Coopersmith Self-Esteem Inventory, semi-structured interview and observation.

Independent variable: The protocol designed using hypnosis as a psychotherapeutic method. Elements of Rational Emotive Behavioral Therapy, Solution Focused Brief Therapy and Transpersonal Psychotherapy of Emotive Expression and Imagery were integrated. The fundamental therapeutic resources proposed were regression, progression, metaphors of protection and change, imagery, autoscopy and hypnobiodramaturgy.

Techniques and Procedures:

The research consisted of three stages:

Diagnostic Stage.

During this stage, the selected persons were visited and asked for informed consent, their agreement to participate in all research activities was recorded, and a battery of specific psychological tests was applied to measure the manifestations associated with suicidal behavior: anxiety and depression as well as self-esteem.

Intervention Stage.

Once the preceding stage was completed, the protocol designed for the treatment of suicidal behavior in adolescence based on the application of hypnosis was applied.

Evaluative Stage.

Two months after the end of the sessions, the same battery of tests was applied to measure the dependent variable and the associated alterations. In both measurements (diagnostic and evaluative stage), double-blind measurements were performed. The double-blind method is a tool of the scientific method used to prevent the results of an investigation from being influenced by the placebo effect or observer bias.

Data collection, processing and analysis techniques.

The information collected through the techniques applied before and after the intervention was processed in computerized form using the McNemar statistical test. The data were processed on a microcomputer using Excel for Windows. The results were expressed in text and tables.

Description of the techniques and tests used.

-Inventory of Trait-State Anxiety (IDARE): Authors: C. D. Spielberger, R. L. Gorsuch, R. E. Lushene. Description: The IDARE is a self-assessing inventory designed to assess two relatively independent forms of anxiety: anxiety as a state (transient emotional condition) and anxiety as a trait (relatively stable anxious propensity), self-administered. Each has 20 items. In the IDARE, there are 10 positive anxiety items (i.e., the higher the score, the higher the anxiety) and 10 negative items. In the trait scale there are 13 positive and 7 negative items. The response form ranges from 0 to 4 in both subscales.

In the State Scale, the subject is oriented to answer how he/she feels at the present moment in relation to the formulated items, and how he/she feels generally in relation to the items of the Trait Anxiety Scale. There are different Spanish versions of the test, one of the most widely used being that of Ch. Spielberger, R. Díaz Guerrero et al (1966), which is the one we use in Cuba.

Validation in Cuba was carried out in 1986 by Castellanos, Grau and Martín. Since then, it has been used in daily care in almost all health institutions in the country, as well as in teaching and research.

-<u>Trait-State Depression Inventory (IDERE):</u> It is a test to study the presence or absence of depression. It consists of a self-assessment inventory divided into two parts *(Grau, Martín, Ramírez, 1989)*. Designed to assess two relatively independent forms of depression: depression as a state (transient emotional condition) and depression as a trait (propensity to suffer depressive states as a relatively stable personality quality).

The scale that evaluates depression as a state allows rapid identification of people who have depressive symptoms, as well as feelings of sadness reactive to situations of loss or threat, which are not necessarily structured as a depressive disorder, although they cause discomfort and disability.

It has 20 items whose answers take values from 1 to 4. Half of these items, due to their content, are positive in depressive states, while the other half are items antagonistic to depression. The subject must select the alternative that best describes his or her state at that moment and has four response options: Not at all (worth 1 point), A little (worth 2 points), Quite a lot (worth 3 points) and A lot (worth 4 points).

The trait depression scale allows the identification of patients who are prone to depressive states and also provides information on the stability of depressive symptoms.

It consists of 22 items that also acquire values from 1 to 4 points and the response options are: Almost Never (worth 1 point), Sometimes (worth 2 points), Frequently (3 points) and Almost Always (4 points).

The values range from 20 to 80 points for the state scale and 20 to 88 points for the trait scale.

Coopersmith's self-esteem inventory: This questionnaire was developed by Coopersmith based on studies carried out in the area of self-esteem. Its objective is to determine the level of self-esteem of individuals and it is made up of 25 propositions (items) where the subject must respond affirmatively or negatively.

A point is awarded in those items that are written in a positive sense and to which the subject answers "yes", these items are: 1, 4, 5, 8, 9, 14, 19, 20. When the subject answers "no", in the remaining items a point is given in the score of that item. At the end, these scores are added together to obtain a total score. The use of this inventory in Mental Health services in Cuba is validated by MINSAP, and this result is interpreted from a norm of percentiles made to classify the subjects according to three levels:

a) High level of self-esteem:

Subjects classified at this level score between 19 and 24 points. They obtain points in most of the items that indicate happiness, efficiency, self-confidence, autonomy, emotional stability, favorable interpersonal relationships, express uninhibited behavior in a group, without focusing on themselves or their own problems.

b) Medium level of self-esteem:

The subjects classified in this level are those who score between 13 and 18 points. They present characteristics of the high and low levels, with no predominance of one level over the other.

c) Low level of self-esteem:

Subjects in this group score less than 12 points. They obtain few points in the items that indicate adequate self-esteem and that were described above. In this sense, subjects at this level perceive themselves as unhappy, insecure, focused on themselves and their particular problems, fearful of expressing themselves in groups, where their emotional state depends on external values and demands.

Interview: Because the psychological interview is considered a clinical technique par excellence. This cannot be absent in the assessment of the subjects studied. It is applied with defined objectives for which questions are asked in relation to suicidal behavior and associated alterations, previously raised.

The thematic content is present in the interview, which is nothing more than the issues that are discussed in relation to suicidal behavior. A balance is evaluated between the ideas that are addressed and the feelings that are manifested in the subject's behavior. Coherence in relation to the orientation given to the issues addressed due to the intensity of the response elaborated by the evaluee and the concurrence of the ideas.

Observation: The guide used evaluates facial expression that explains mood, as well as posture, work rhythm, behavior before the applied techniques of evaluation and treatment, the elements proper to oral expression in terms of: volume, speed, tone. The physical appearance of the evaluated subject and the attitude manifested before the evaluator. Observation as a resource is implicit at all times in the development of the research.

form
HYPNOTHERAPEUTIC PROTOCOL FOR SUICIDAL BEHAVIOR IN ADOLESCENCE

STAGES OF THE PROTOCOL:

(Four stages, the first two being the first session)

1. Identify suicidal behavior according to:

    - Informed consent (Annex 1)

    - Category in which it is expressed (suicidal ideation, suicidal threat, suicidal attempt).

    - Criminalize the conduct if the suicide attempt has been made.

    - Identify capacities and abilities (Capacities: Set of individual psychological peculiarities that respond to socially stable activities) (Abilities: Facility for the execution of the activity that is developed with the exercise).

    - Identify the stage of development of the subject under study: Crisis, communication and activity system, significant experiences as a unit of analysis of the social situation of development.

2. Therapeutic contract.

- Measurement of the dependent variable:

  suicidal behavior and anxiety-depression as associated disorders.

Techniques to be used in the first and last measurement: IDARE, IDERE, Interview, Observation.

- Discussion of myths about hypnosis.

<u>Is hypnosis related to magic, spiritualism and the possibility of returning to past lives?</u>

The hypnotic *state* has absolutely nothing to do with illusionism or necromancy, its regularities as a scientific fact do not share any characteristics with them, although it has often been presented in this guise in public spectacles for profit. The beliefs of the subject determine in a qualitative sense the intrahypnotic experiences.

<u>Can you hypnotize a person by snapping your fingers or staring at them?</u>

The spectacular results produced by the use of these methods have nothing to do with black magic, far from it, although there is nothing to do with charlatanism and lack of ethics.

They are based on the conditioning that occurs during the hypnotic process, in which an intentional associative connection can be established between any clue and the special *state* of consciousness that is reached (sign signal), then the conditioning continues to occur under the unique neurophysiological conditions of the new *state* reached, which is strongly anchored to the pre-established symbol, whether it is a phrase, a snap of the fingers, or a way of staring into the eyes.

<u>Do people who engage in hypnosis have supernatural gifts to totally dominate the hypnotized person?</u>

In the movies, and in the spectacular demonstrations exploited by the media, the protagonists create the illusion that they possess a supernatural magical force over other people, hence the emergence of this myth that has been reinforced by the surprising objective manifestations of hypnosis for which no neuropsychological explanation is given.

<u>Are some people easier to hypnotize than others?</u>

Potentially anyone can be hypnotized, even seemingly un-suggestible people can experience the state with special techniques up to some stage of it.

<u>Does the hypnotic *state* only occur in people who are easy to dominate?</u>

All normal people have their temperament, character and personality, so they can experience, to some degree and nuance, hypnotic-like phenomena without being formally hypnotized, of course with the contextual location and logical differences involving different situations, so that the unusual would be a person completely incapable of experiencing these phenomena.

<u>Can the person come out of the hypnotic *state* at any time he/she wishes?</u>
If the patient decides to interrupt the hypnotic process, he/she can do so of his/her own free will in the initial stages, but in order to do so in deeper stages, the therapist must have indicated this in the content of his/her suggestions, and he/she must have specified the freedom to leave the *state* at any time during the process.

This last type of permissive suggestion is of transcendental ethical importance, so it is necessary to keep in mind, once again, that the nature of the hypnotic process is always contextually determined, and that the content of the suggestions and the degree of depth determine many things.

<u>Once the hypnotic *state* has been experienced, can the person not avoid being hypnotized thereafter?</u>
The main cause of the emergence of the belief that one loses the will to refuse to undergo hypnosis again, once one has gone through the process before, is the scientifically proven existence of the *signal sign*, which consists of a type of suggestion that is reinforced during previous hypnotic processes and which effectively serves for a very rapid re-

induction that avoids the initial stages of the process, so that the patient passes instantly to the very deep stage when the signal sign is suggested without going through the initial stages.

Could the hypnotic *state* be irreversible?

The panic of not being able to come out of the hypnotic *state* possibly originates from the well-known fact that frequently occurs when the specialist offers the alternative of "waking up" the patient or opening his eyes and the patient does not open them for a while.

The answer to the irreversibility of the hypnotic *state* is that it is impossible for a person to remain hypnotized forever. The reasons for this are based on the hypothesis that hypnosis is a mode of waking consciousness in which the brain temporarily functions subconsciously; such a *state* can be reversed with appropriate suggestions or allow the person to evolve spontaneously.

Can the hypnotic *state* cause the hypnotized person to speak what he/she does not want to and do things against his/her will?

Evidently, this is a myth that, in addition to being one of the most frequent, constitutes the expression of the fear of invasion of the privacy of our most reserved thoughts and feelings.

In the clinical context, the specialist offers suggestions that the patient interprets as useful to solve his or her health problem, and therefore accepts them as part of the therapist-patient relationship, in which ethical codes that follow the criteria of good clinical practice and others of a moral nature operate.

In general terms, it must be admitted that people in the hypnotic *state* retain the same capacity to do or say things as in the waking state, but this would only be true if the context and *state* of consciousness that occur in the two states were identical, however, the rules that operate in the hypnotic *state*, in a neuropsychological sense, are different from those of habitual wakefulness.

This determines that the characteristics of the communicative, affective, volitional and cognitive relationship are essentially different in the hypnotic *state*.

In experimental contexts it can be proved that during the hypnotic *state* there is a state logic that determines that the ideation can be channeled towards a certain end.

- Definition of therapeutic objectives per session.
- Duration:

45min/1 hour.

- Frequency of sessions:
  Once a week.

- First neutral induction with utilization.

Essential hypnotic phenomena and their characteristics according to each stage or degree of depth.

1. *Very mild or hypnoidal stage*

   Muscle relaxation, general heaviness and eyelid closure.

2. *Mild Stage*

   Catalepsy of the eyelids and catalepsy of the limbs.

3. *Middle Stage*

   General catalepsy, suggested automatic movements, sleep suggestions, deepening techniques, the sign signal is applied for the first time.

4. *Deep Stage*

Superficial anesthesia, Sensory disturbances, Simple post-hypnotic suggestions, Auditory, gustatory and olfactory hallucinations, Conversation without awakening, Partial amnesia

5. *Very deep stage*

Opening the eyes without going out of state, Complicated hallucinations, Age regressions, Behavior with state logic according to suggestions (literalness), Complicated post-hypnotic suggestions, Complicated post-hypnotic hallucinations, Deep anesthesia, Deep amnesia

3. Individualized hypnotherapeutic sessions according to subjects, adjusting to the exclusive use of protocolized techniques.

   The stages of anchoring (throughout the therapeutic process)
   a) The subject is asked to recall a moment in life when we acted in an exceptional way that we would like to repeat in any new situation.
   b) You are asked to relive the past experience with all your senses,

until you feel it intensely. This implies seeing, hearing, feeling, etc. in fullness.

c) You are asked to find a place on your body to store that experience, for example the knuckles of your hands or your right ear.

d) You are asked to place a finger on the right knuckle or ear to install the anchor. With eyes closed, the experience should be perceived in a state of concentration for a few seconds.

e) Quality control. Test daily whether placing the finger on the knuckle or ear reproduces the experience, if not, calibrate until this is achieved.

f) A successful anchor is the beginning, many more resources can be added to be available when the situation requires it.

g) Learning to anchor oneself to the best moments and the best responses is learning to draw resources from an internal battery that recharges with each experience. Learning to use the brain is much better than leaving it on autopilot because we can give it direction.

3.1 <u>Symptomatological suppression:</u>(second session)

Anxiety is suppressed by the state of progressive relaxation conditioned by the suggestions of the very mild or hypnoidal state, which is guaranteed by the technique of body scanning whose method is to suggest progressive relaxation from the feet to the head by muscle groups. In a second moment in the mild stage, it is suggested to the subject to build a safe place or safe harbor where he/she feels completely protected, relaxed and calm.

Depression as a state is suppressed with the use of process suggestions in a mild and medium hypnotic state and is indicated through the use of metaphorical language and the construction of protective symbols that increase self-esteem, control and security.

The hypnotic state as a submodality of the waking state has the singularity of inhibiting the past-future psychological times, thus guaranteeing a contextualization in the present time, in this way it works for regressions and age progressions where the subject does not remember but lives the intra-hypnotic experience.

It highlights the impossibility of manifesting depression and anxiety due to the temporary contents from the psychological point of view inherent to each of these emotional responses that they encompass:

Subjective or cognitive aspects of unpleasant character, bodily or physiological aspects characterized by a high degree of activation of the peripheral system, observable or motor aspects that usually involve poorly adjusted and poorly adaptive behaviors.

3.2 <u>Behavioral</u> modification <u>specific to suicidal behavior</u> (Third session).

Use of reinforcement in each of the subsequent sessions, using therapeutic resources such as summation.

Rational emotive behavioral therapy:

The model has been continuously expanded to meet the needs of clinical practice. According to Lega, Caballo and Ellis (1997)

A (Observed events)

B ("Beliefs": Interpretations and value judgments, about A)

- rB: Rational beliefs
- iB: Irrational beliefs

C (Consequences of beliefs B on events A)

- Ced: Desired emotional consequences
- Ccd: Desired behavioral outcomes
- Cei: Undesirable emotional consequences
- Cci: Undesirable Behavioral Consequences

D (Debate or rational questioning process)

- Efcg: Cognitive strategies (Socratic dialogue, bibliotherapy, and others).
- Efe: Emotional Strategies (trials through imagination)
- Efc: Behavioral strategies (empirical reality testing and behavioral trials)

E (Effects of the questioning process and practice)

<u>Intrahypnotic application:</u>

A: Definition of the experience that according to the personal sense of the particular subject conditions suicidal behavior.

B: Identify the subject's specific knowledge in particular about the risk factors associated with suicidal behavior, complications, consequences, lethality of the method used and intentionality of dying with the behavior manifested.

C: To identify the belief systems socially acquired by the subject that lead to suicidal behavior as a way out of the situation defined as problematic.

D: Discussion of irrational ideas with the intention of achieving homogenization in the affective-cognitive-behavioral components. The use of solution-focused coping mechanisms is ensured.

E: Effects of the questioning process according to the construction of scenarios where healthy behavior is manifested and consequences are described in practice. Cognitive reconfiguration of the event and alternatives to propose solutions.

<u>Therapeutic sessions using complicated intrahypnotic suggestions.</u>

(Fourth, fifth and sixth sessions)

Objective: Symptomatological suppression associated with alterations in the content of thought: overvalued ideas, suicidal ideas and anhedonia as a qualitative symptom of the affective sphere evident in moderate and deep depressions.

Techniques:

The techniques used are built through imagery where symbols are developed and specific resources are applied: empty chair, hyperthermia, regressions and progressions and hypnobiodramaturgy.

Flowers and thorns: The clients in vigil are asked to describe or characterize a flower, let's say a rose. The beauty of roses is highlighted and how, together with such beauty, there are thorns that hurt, hurt but also protect. Life is like a very beautiful rose but it always has its thorns.

- Progressive relaxation is induced, combined with breathing.

- The modulation of the tone of the voice is important; in an energetic way but in a low tone, the beautiful shades of life are accentuated, such as the color of your preference expressed in a flower. Keeping the tone low and slightly rising, the existence of thorns is recognized as a synonym of discomfort, pain, difficulties, failures.

- Suggestions are made to mean that despite the thorns, roses are increasingly accepted for the beauty of its different shapes, colors, which can change in every season of the year...... As the pain that are thorns, are present, but never minimize the beauty of the rose, roses and thorns always together inseparable, expression of love, defense and protection....

- Breathing away my pain(emtional): Hypnotic induction by progressive relaxation, partial breathing (abdominal) and then complete breathing (abdominal - thoracic) are performed.

- When the patient is in a medium to deep hypnotic state, he is instructed to locate his pain and mentally describe it.

- Suggestion of experiencing the presence of pain that is present in time and body space... well localized... or as far as it radiates... slowly... as a beam of light becomes fainter... fainter and fainter....

- The image or memory of a beautiful river is represented, the subject with his back to it... and as if he throws towards the waters... that run, moving further and further away... his pain... as he relaxes more and more... it moves further away, much further away, completely imperceptible ......

Flood of light: It refers to the body being flooded by a beam of very faint green light (the color depends on the identification of the subject), which is healing and increasingly approaches the affected area. It is important that the patient is persuaded of his pain (emotional), recognize it and discard it, through therapeutic suggestions.

- It is suggested that you represent what your grief is like, locate it, define it, identify it and slowly you perceive that it is moving away, that it is moving away from you, at least it is becoming more pleasant, more tolerant.

- To prepare the patient for his exit from the state, in a natural way and some post-hypnotic suggestion can be added to him to be carried out at home, at bedtime or at the beginning of the day or during the day when he feels discomfort or to prevent these discomforts.

The Empty Chair technique:

(*empty chair* has been commonly associated with the practice of Gestalt therapy, it basically consists of mentally creating a character with which one wants to confront a problem, then assuming his role in his place and then answering in the subject's place with the role that belongs to himself).

It is the basic element for the therapeutic work in this approach. It basically consists of highlighting the person's internal dialogue. In this dialogue, in Perls' terms, the "top dog" and the "bottom dog" confront each other; that is to say, everything by which we feel oppressed (as a result of the introjects) and the role with which we have identified ourselves as victims ("bottom dog"). In practice, this top dog can be represented by the father, mother, boss, friends, partner, etc.

During therapy, different meanings can be given to the same uses as with the *hot chair*, the subject moves from one chair to another, represents each of the roles and expresses his emotions, so that, wherever he is, all the ideas and feelings are the patient's own. In this way the main objective of the *chair* is achieved, which is the collection of the projection and the closure of the situation.

Hyperthermia in the therapeutic process

Focus attention on the voice and provoke a feeling of relaxation in the whole body as is done in any hypnotic induction.

A zone induction is performed to focus the attention on the specific location to be worked on. The neighboring organs should be protected in the work with suggestions that condition this, then the hyperconcentration on the treated organ or part should be intensified (the subject is always instructed to point out or identify an area where emotions and feelings are expressed).

The patient must know everything that is happening or should happen during the therapy, e.g.: in these moments the negative emotions-feelings dissolve, evaporate and your "liver regenerates and recovers its normal state and appearance".

The most successful suggestions are of a meadow-forest-field; it is suggested that he walks, smells, feels, enjoys the landscape and at the entrance of the forest it is suggested that he asks a question that conditions an answer to his particular situations... the objective is to open the emotional expression that accompanies the (psychological) lesion that is the reason for the consultation.

Start with therapeutic work with self-esteem and self-control with countdown to deepen state.

A reciprocal inhibitor is installed (place or safe harbor, particular place of the subject, he is told that it is a place that allows him to feel extremely relaxed...) a count of 3, 2, 1 is made and he is instructed to swallow saliva, thus dissociating him or distracting him cognitively. This is done because symptoms with overflowing emotional content distort the patient's real situation.

It is performed according to the need for glandular stimulation by autoscopy (thyroid, lymphocytes, NK cells, macrophages, etc.).

<u>Metaphors to use</u>

A dwarf with a blowtorch or fire gun is able to burn and stop the growth of negative emotions-feelings, malignant or bad, all depending on the cultural level of the patient.

An erupting volcano that is very powerful where the damaged area is dropped in the center of the volcano so that the burning lava burns everything that harms the patient's health.

Suggestions of regeneration of the area, taking into account that the patient may believe that the whole organ was damaged by the fire so it is necessary to regenerate it to bring it to the normal anatomical-functional state. Example areas where there are mucous membranes, an autoscopy metaphor is used where the organ is invaded by an army of little white men (it is explained that it is the immune system).

Some finish eliminating the malignant cells-emotions-feelings that may remain, others throw away the waste and others reconstruct the organ as it was before getting sick.... which conditions an affective state that adjusts the healthy manifestations of the subject's behaviors.

1.3. <u>Personological modification specific to suicidal behavior.</u>

(Sessions seven-eight)

Objective: To condition the behavioral stability of the health-oriented subject in any context where the behavior is manifested.

Resources to be used:

Use of Transpersonal Psychotherapy strategies of Emotional Expression and Imagery.

Impermanence: Everything exists in a time limit, even time itself, for those of us who perceive it at some point in our lives we will stop doing it. Each stage of life (childhood, adolescence, youth and adulthood) and the physical characteristics inherent to each of them are also, condition the possibility that everything that happens as they begin and end, are good or bad according to the personal evaluations of each person in a specific situation.

Ex: Life is like reading a book, it becomes necessary to turn the page to finish each chapter, the end of it does not necessarily mean that the book is over but that each time it is more interesting, things happen that we do not think, just to keep us in a comfort zone that prevents us from enjoying the next page, maybe…, a new chapter….

Detachment: Once we have understood Impermanence as a concept we can identify the need to detach ourselves from each event in our lives, this does not mean thinking that nothing is important but contrary to this, it should only have the temporary importance necessary to give an answer. Prior to this we must know if it has one.

Is the problem I identify mine? To what extent does it depend on me? Does it have a solution? Am I responsible for providing it? Is it really a problem? Detachment means depositing sufficient energy not in the final objective or goal but in the process itself.

Ex: Sometimes when we start a relationship, one of the partners asks a common question: Will it last forever?

In order to know how long we will last in terms of relationship, we must know that it is not more important how much we do but what we do so that this end is consolidated, that is, the process itself. The possibility of voluntarily using psychological times without this conditioning a pathological emotional state such as anxiety or depression.

The proper use of time means a permanence in the present, with the search in the past for valuable resources that condition success, from the design of scenarios where our behavior is contextualized with a healthy perspective.

<u>Intrahypnotic techniques:</u>

In each session, the achievements obtained in each of the stages must be reinforced in order to guarantee therapeutic success.

Age progressions:

Possible scenarios where the subject's behavior manifests itself in a healthy way are identified.

To be able to know oneself once the expected state of pleasant health has been achieved.

Identify situations that may have generated a conflict in the past, or may exist in the future.

To achieve alternatives of confrontation from an affective state that in cognitive balance focuses the patient's behavior on solutions.

In this way, a subject is achieved who, from the understanding of the emotions that emanate from the situation defined as a problem, builds healthy solutions contrary to the self-destructive behaviors that generated the reason for the initial consultation.

4. Closing the therapeutic relationship:

- The patient is discharged once compliance with the therapeutic objectives has been assessed.

- Establish the possibility of returning to consultation when deemed convenient, even knowing as a therapist that one of the aspects to be taken into account from the ethical point of view is to guarantee the therapeutic independence of the subject-client-patient.

- Appointment for measurement of the identified variables three months after discharge (Suicidal Behavior, Self-Esteem, Anxiety and Depression).

The definition of eight therapeutic sessions as a proposal for the established protocol does not mean that a readjustment for the particularities of the subject is denied. The use of each resource as determined in the methodology of the present Hypnotherapeutic Protocol for Suicidal Behavior in Adolescence <u>is mandatory</u>.

Specialist Criteria:
The methodology designed in the protocol proposed in the study was used to triangulate, taking into account the assessment of specialists in the field of hypnosis in Cuba and Chile.

- DrC. Alberto Erconvaldo Cobián Mena.

Doctor in Psychological Sciences. President of the Cuban Society of Health Psychology. Founding President of the Panamerican and Caribbean Association of Therapeutic Hypnosis.

Agrees with the methodological structure according to the fulfillment of the proposed psychotherapeutic objectives. Proposes to add the explanation of the use of Rational Emotive Behavioral Psychotherapy in hypnotic state.

- Dr. Cristobal Schilling Fuenzalida.

Specialist in Clinical Psychology. Director of the Clinical Hypnosis Center of Chile. Secretary of the Panamerican and Caribbean Association of Therapeutic Hypnosis.

Proposes to describe the proposed techniques and the content of the metaphors used. It agrees with the use of the principles of Impermanence and Detachment from the Transpersonal Psychotherapy of Emotive Expression and Imagery.

- DrC. Pedro Manuel Rodríguez Sánchez.

Doctor in Medical Sciences. Second Degree Specialist in Normal and Pathological Physiology. Vice President of the Panamerican and Caribbean Association of Therapeutic Hypnosis.

It agrees with the definition of hypnosis proposed to support the use of this technique as a psychotherapeutic tool in the designed protocol.

He proposes to point out the eminently psychological induction to the hypnotic state and the position as a scientist on Hypnosis and its classification as a submodality of the waking state in the definition proposed for the Doctoral Thesis "Neurophysiological Foundations of Hypnosis".

SIGNIFICANT RESULTS

The manifestation of the levels of expression of anxiety as a trait state in the sample subjects before and after the treatment protocol was applied.

For trait and state, a high level was obtained (60% and 89.3%) before treatment. Once concluded and evaluated according to the guidelines defined in the protocol, a significant decrease to a low level was observed for trait (91%) and state (97%) of the sample studied.

When evaluating the results according to McNemar, it is evident that the protocol achieves significant transformations in the subjects as the calculated chi-square values for trait (67.7) and state (134.8) exceed the tabulated chi-square values (5.99) for two degrees of freedom and p≤0.05.

Collings S, Jenkin G, Stanley J, McKenzie S, Hatcher S,[25] in investigations carried out with the application of different treatment methods for suicidal behavior in adolescence obtain results below those obtained in the present study even when the associated alterations are evaluated by means of other types of tests.

Urrego Betancourt Y,[35] shows figures lower than 90% of the research sample in the levels of expression of anxiety as a trait-state. The consistent difference is given in the particularities of the study and the methodology used for the measurement of the evaluated affective state.

Anxiety and depression are a set of responses that include: subjective or cognitive aspects of unpleasant character, bodily or physiological aspects characterized by a high degree of activation of the peripheral system, observable or motor aspects that usually involve poorly adjusted and poorly adaptive behaviors, as Martín Pérez V. points out. [53]

The relevance of the study according to the results observable in this table, in the author's opinion, is given by the specificity and precision of the measurement before and after the intervention, which does not leave room for speculation.

The reading of the protocol and the methodological structure required for its application, allows the therapist to know the stability of the changes. The definition of psychotherapeutic objectives allows the suppression of the referred symptomatology, the modification of the behavior before the situation that triggers the behavior and the re-education of the personality that allows a structured regulation of the behavior of the treated subjects.

This conditions that the proposed protocol, in addition to being unique in the context where it is applied, is effective as demonstrated by the statistical processing of the results achieved in the research sample. These criteria coincide with Pérez Almoza, G. Bestard Bizet, R.S. [46]

Once the designed protocol was applied, it can be seen that the levels of depression as a trait-state decreased significantly. Before the treatment 57% of the sample had a high level of depression as a trait and 92% as a state. Once the protocol was applied, 93% of the sample had a low level of depression as a trait and 99% had a low level of depression as a state. This demonstrates the effectiveness of the protocol in the subjects of the sample studied.

When evaluating the results according to McNemar, it is evident that the protocol determines significant changes in the subjects since the chi-square values calculated for trait (125.08) and state (142.72) exceed the tabulated chi-square values (5.99) for two degrees of freedom and $p \leq 0.05$.

It is valid to point out that the permanence in the medium level of depression as a 7% trait is given by the stability of personality traits. Subjects who experience negative affective states such as anxiety and depression in a prolonged manner over time, make apprehension of the symptom and it is incorporated as part of the structure of the personality, in this way the total possibility of modification becomes complex, according to Darke S, Cambell G, Popple G.[22]

Sandoval Ato R, Vilela Estrada MA, Galvez Olortegui J,[32] achieved modifications in the levels of depression that allow the individual to function in an adequate way, which allows an adaptation to the demands of the environment without psychopathological manifestations. The most significant data is the decrease in the low level of depression as a state trait in 87 and 93%. These data are significant for their research sample. The results obtained in the current research differ from the previous ones by a difference of 5 and 6% for the studied sample.

No records were found in the literature of treatments with large samples such as the present study of the application of hypnosis in patients with suicidal behavior where depression is an associated disorder.

Only in the single case study published by Pérez Almoza G,[18] where the result obtained before the application of hypnosis as a therapeutic resource was high levels of depression as a trait-state, after the treatment a decrease of the trait to medium level was obtained, and as a state depression decreased to low level.

The second measurement of depression levels was performed six months after the last therapeutic session with the intention of demonstrating the stability of the results achieved after the intervention. [18]

According to the author of the present study, the protocol designed and applied, in addition to being novel in its methodological structure and therapeutic proposal, is effective for the research sample. The results obtained show the possibility of standardizing the proposal for the treatment of suicidal behavior in adolescence.

The psychotherapeutic approach using hypnosis modifies the expression of self-esteem levels before and after the intervention. 68% of the research sample showed low levels of self-esteem, only 4% of the sample showed a high level. Afterwards, a significant increase of 93% to a high level was observed, and only 4% of the sample persisted in a low level of self-esteem with 3 subjects of the total studied.

When determining the inferential statistics, calculated values of chi-square according to McNemar for self-esteem were 119.86, which exceed the tabulated values for two degrees of freedom and probability less than or equal to 0.05, so it can be affirmed that the results are statistically significant.

As this is the first time that a protocol based on Hypnosis for the treatment of suicidal behavior in adolescence has been designed and applied in Cuba, it is not possible to identify previous records to make comparisons of divergence and convergence, this, until the moment of consultation of the international bibliography for the development of the research.

Authors such as Dedić G,[24] and Martín Pérez, V,[53] have developed programs, strategies and protocols to intervene in suicidal behavior with the aim of identifying or characterizing it. There are few traces of demonstrated effectiveness in the designs and application of these with discrete results, 67% of the sample increased levels of self-esteem in the first, the second is limited to the description of the protocol without evidence of its application in defined samples that affirm some kind of effectiveness.

It should be noted that the evaluation of self-esteem was based on the design and application of surveys that were not validated or contrasted with the criteria of specialists in the field of Mental Health, Suicidal Behavior and the study of Self-Esteem.[24]

The results achieved coincide with Sandoval-Ato R, Vilela-Estrada MA, Galvez-Olortegui J,[31] who studied a smaller sample and a different intervention proposal with the aim of modifying knowledge about suicidal behavior and its risk factors. The main result with which the present study agrees is the increase in knowledge about high self-esteem as a protective factor; 95% of the sample showed adequate knowledge on this subject.

The study by Pineda MS, Matos Premiot JY, Heredia Barroso D,[29] aimed at the modification of knowledge or identification of consequences of self-destructive behaviors such as suicidal behavior, is limited to the instruction of the subjects who participate in these; not so for the modification of behaviors as genesis of health, or the personological restructuring that evidences an adequate level of regulation that orients the behavior to the well-being and adaptation to the demands of the environment, according to the author's criteria.

With the results obtained, it can be concluded that once the proposed protocol was designed and applied, there is a female supremacy in the subjects of the sample studied. The predominant age group is 15-19 years old and the race is white; the triggering vital event is the family conflict with the method of ingestion of tablets. For this study, religiosity and personal history of previous suicide attempts are not elements to be taken into account as risk or protective factors. The protocol is effective for the treatment of suicidal behavior as a reason for consultation, increases the levels of self-esteem and decreases anxiety and depression as alterations associated with suicidal behavior.

Main Statistics

Anxiety	Levels	Formerly No.	%	Then No.	%
Feature	High	45	60	-	-
	Medium	27	36	7	9
	Under	3	4	68	91
State	High	67	89,3	-	-
	Medium	7	9,3	2	3
	Under	1	1,3	73	97

Depression	Levels	Formerly No.	%	Then No.	%
Feature	High	43	57	-	-
	Medium	30	40	5	7
	Under	2	3	70	93
State	High	69	92	-	-
	Medium	5	7	1	1
	Under	1	1	74	99

Self-esteem	Formerly No.	%	Then No.	%
High level	3	4	70	93
Medium level	21	28	2	3
Low level	51	68	3	4
Total	75	100	75	100

GABRIEL PÉREZ ALMOZA

BIBLIOGRAPHY CONSULTED

Cruz Rodríguez E, Moreira Ríos I, Orraca Castillo O, Pérez Morino N, Hernández Gonzales P. Risk factors for suicide attempts in adolescents. Rev Cienc Med December 2011; 15 (4).

García Santiesteban JL, Piñeda Ramírez A, Almaguer Brito L. Suicide attempt and adolescence: A theoretical look at the phenomenon. Rev Electron 2011; 36(1). Available at: <http://www.ltu.sld.cu/revista/modules.php?name=News&file=article&sid=186/es> [accessed: 11 January 2015].

Soler Santana R, Castillo Núñez B, Brossard Cisneros M. Quality in the execution of the Suicidal Behavior Prevention and Control Program. MEDISAN 2010; 14(5). Accessed: 11 January 2015. Available at: http://bvs.sld.cu/revistas/san/vol_14_5_10/san10510.htm

Martínez Sedeño, Ávila Aveleira. Behavior of the Suicide Attempt in the municipality of Manatí during 2007 and 2008. VOL. 35 NO. 1 YEAR. 14 January-March 2010. [accessed17/1/2015] Available at: http://www.ltu.sld.cu/revista/modules.php?name=News&file=article&sid=55

Suicide attempt as a cause of intoxication in pediatrics. Revista Cubana de Medicina Intensiva y Emergencias 2007;6(4).Accessed: 25-2-2015. Available at: http://bvs.sld.cu/revistas/mie/vol6_4_07/mie08407.htm

Suicide attempt behavior in the municipality of nueva paz. Revista de Ciencias Médicas La Habana 2008; 14 (3),[Consulted: 25-2-2015] Available at: http://www.cpicmha.sld.cu/hab/vol14_3_08/hab02308.html

Bibliomed on depression and suicide attempt. Rev. Cubana Med Gen Integr 2007; 23(1). Accessed: 22 January 2018. Available at: <http://scielo.sld.cu/scielo.php?script=sci_arttext&pid=S08641252007000100021&lng=es&nrm=iso>

Elba Vázquez P, Ignacio Fonseca C, Juan Ramón Padilla V. Diagnosis of depression in suicidal and healthy adolescents. Bol Clin Hosp Infant Edo Son 2008. 22(2) 107-118.

Mislay Rodríguez G, Deisy Boris S, Omar Rodríguez O. Some epidemiological aspects of depression in the elderly. MEDISAN 2011; 13(5).

Oliva Martínez M. Behavior of suicidal behavior in the municipality of San José de Las Lajas. Revista Ciencias Médicas La Habana 2009; 13(2).

Trenzado Rodríguez N, Canosa Besu LB, González Pérez H. Epidemiology of suicide in Cárdenas. Rev. medica electron 20010; 30(4). [Accessed: 1 March 2015]. Available at: http://www.revmatanzas.sld.cu/revista%20medica/ano%202008/vol4%202008/tema01.htm

www.ingramcontent.com/pod-product-compliance
Lightning Source LLC
Chambersburg PA
CBHW071057240526
45471CB00016B/1973